# A-Z of
## Complementary and
## Alternative Medicine

Commissioning Editor: *Claire Wilson*
Development Editor: *Kerry McGechie/Veronika Watkins*
Project Manager: *Joannah Duncan*
Designer: *Charles Gray*

# A-Z of
# Complementary and Alternative Medicine

## A GUIDE FOR HEALTH PROFESSIONALS

## Fiona Mantle RN RHV Cert Ed. RNT

*Staff Nurse, John Radcliffe Hospital, Oxford; freelance writer and lecturer in complementary and alternative medicine*

## Denise Tiran MSc RM RGN ADM PGCEA

*Director, Expectancy Ltd, London; Visiting Lecturer, University of Greenwich, London; lecturer and practitioner in complementary medicine*

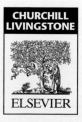

CHURCHILL
LIVINGSTONE

ELSEVIER

Edinburgh   London   New York   Oxford   Philadelphia   St Louis   Sydney   Toronto   2009

# CHURCHILL
# LIVINGSTONE
### ELSEVIER

© 2009, Elsevier Limited. All rights reserved.

ISBN: 978-0-443-10329-2

**British Library Cataloguing in Publication Data**
A catalogue record for this book is available from the British Library

**Library of Congress Cataloging in Publication Data**
A catalog record for this book is available from the Library of Congress

## Notice

Knowledge and best practice in this field are constantly changing. As new research and experience broaden our knowledge, changes in practice, treatment and drug therapy may become necessary or appropriate. Readers are advised to check the most current information provided (i) on procedures featured or (ii) by the manufacturer of each product to be administered, to verify the recommended dose or formula, the method and duration of administration, and contraindications. It is the responsibility of the practitioner, relying on their own experience and knowledge of the patient, to make diagnoses, to determine dosages and the best treatment for each individual patient, and to take all appropriate safety precautions. To the fullest extent of the law, neither the Publisher nor the Editors assume any liability for any injury and/or damage to persons or property arising out or related to any use of the material contained in this book. It is the responsibility of the treating practitioner, relying on independent expertise and knowledge of the patient, to determine the best treatment and method of application for the patient.

*The Publisher*

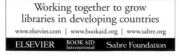

ELSEVIER · your source for books, journals and multimedia in the health sciences

**www.elsevierhealth.com**

Working together to grow libraries in developing countries
www.elsevier.com | www.bookaid.org | www.sabre.org
ELSEVIER · BOOK AID International · Sabre Foundation

The Publisher's policy is to use **paper manufactured from sustainable forests**

Printed in China

# Contents

## Breathwork therapies 55

## Cancer therapies 59

## Diagnostic techniques 74

## Other therapies      215

## Relaxation therapies      226

## Traditional systems of medicine      234

# Preface

The last 20 years have witnessed a phenomenal rise in interest in complementary and alternative medicine (CAM), both within the healthcare professions and among the general population, and the Prince of Wales's Foundation for Integrated Health has put CAM firmly on the public and political agenda. Many healthcare professionals have trained in CAM and, with varying degrees of success, have integrated them into clinical practice across a wide range of clinical specialities. It is perhaps due only to lack of information and, more recently, to professional concerns over the evidence base of CAM that precludes a wider use, especially as both the general public and conventional healthcare professionals do not always know where to obtain the most comprehensive and appropriate advice. The use of CAM by individuals appears to result partly from recommendations of family and friends, or through items which prospective users see in the media. Unfortunately, however, health journalists may sometimes be more concerned with product placement than medical accuracy, while some appear to have little or no knowledge about either clinical medicine or the huge range of complementary therapies. This potentially leads to unsafe or inappropriate recommendations and a consequent delay by the public in seeking conventional medical care.

Doctors, nurses and midwives are frequently the first point of contact for people seeking medical help. There is an inherent challenge to accommodate patients and their families who wish to use CAM as part of their healthcare choices, and increasingly, healthcare professionals find themselves being asked for advice and information on some of the alternatives available, particularly since there is a degree of dissatisfaction with certain aspects of National Health Service provision. The role of the healthcare professional encompasses not only the provision of conventional care, but also a duty to provide sufficient information about CAM to enable patients and clients to make informed choices about their healthcare, to promote only those alternative interventions which are proven to be safe and effective and to protect people from dangerous practices and practitioners.

This book aims to offer an introduction to as wide a range of complementary and alternative therapies as possible, including a general description, a brief summary of some of the contemporary evidence, relevant safety issues and contemporary references and resources. The main therapies currently in use in the UK are included, as are many of the more alternative modalities, and some which are more obscure. There are, indeed, several hundred complementary and alternative therapies and the authors acknowledge that certain therapies will have been excluded from this book, which is intended primarily as a 'ready reference' to enable conventional healthcare professionals to access brief information in the clinical setting, provide immediate answers to individual patients or refer them to a more comprehensive source of information.

The therapies are grouped into categories, in alphabetical order, with sub-sections, also alphabetically, covering the individual therapies within the category. Further sub-divisions are used in some sections to explain the terminology and specific elements of a therapy. For example, Chinese medicine is included in the category on Traditional Medicine, with acupuncture being one element of this. By its very nature, the book does not provide an in-depth exploration of each of the therapies, therefore suggestions for further reading are included in the bibliography lists; further supporting evidence can also be obtained from the excellent complementary medicine database at: *http://nccam.nih.gov/camonpubmed/*

# About the Authors

**Fiona Mantle** BSc(Hons) RGN RHV Cert Ed. RNT
*Diploma in Applied Hypnosis, reflex zone therapist; registered Bach flower practitioner; certificate of Homeopathy in Professional Health Care.*

Fiona is an experienced nurse, health visitor and nursing lecturer, now working as a freelance consultant and researcher in complementary medicine. She has written extensively in the nursing press, has presented at national and international conferences, and is the author of a textbook for paediatric nurses, *Complementary and Alternative Medicine for Child and Adolescent Care* (Elsevier 2004). Fiona runs a website for parents who wish to use complementary therapies for their child's health, see: www.naturalchildhealth.co.uk

**Denise Tiran** MSc RM RGN ADM PGCEA
*Director, Expectancy Ltd, London; visiting lecturer, University of Greenwich, London; lecturer and practitioner in complementary medicine.*

Denise is an experienced midwife, complementary practitioner, university lecturer and a renowned international authority in the specialized field of complementary therapies in maternity care. She has written numerous professional textbooks and journal papers, as well as two books for expectant mothers. She is a frequent conference speaker and regularly teaches midwives, doctors and therapists around the UK and overseas. Denise is Director of Expectancy – the Expectant Parents' Complementary Therapies Consultancy – which provides education and consultancy services for professionals, and information and advice for mothers on the safety of complementary therapies in pregnancy and childbirth. See: www.expectancy.co.uk

# Acknowledgements

We are indebted to several people who have kindly given generously of their time and expertise. We would especially like to mention the following individuals at the John Radcliffe Hospital, Oxford: Joan Coleman of the inter-library loans department; Bethan Helby, senior dietician; Victoria Mott, pharmacist in the Drug Information Service, and in particular the helpful and efficient staff of the Cairns Library. We are also grateful for the assistance of: Geraldine Walker and Meryl Burleigh of the Chartered Society of Physiotherapists; Trudy Norris from the National Institute of Medical Herbalists; Dr Michael Heap at Sheffield University and the British Society for Experimental and Clinical Hypnosis; and Professor Peter Molan, Director of the Honey Research Unit at Waikato University in New Zealand.

Fiona would particularly like to acknowledge the help of her mother, Lilian, who gave many wise suggestions for the original text, but who sadly died before publication.

# Dedications

This book is dedicated to Fiona's parents, Lilian and Christopher Mantle, with love and gratitude, and to her dear sister Andrea for her continuing love and support. Denise wishes to dedicate the book to her son, Adam, and her partner, Harry, for their love and patience, as always, while working on the book.

# A

## Animal-assisted therapies

*Description*

Therapies involving animals are particularly beneficial for people with learning or physical disabilities, as well as the elderly and those in long-term residential healthcare settings. While it is acknowledged that animals have been used for relaxation purposes, e.g. swimming with dolphins, these activities have not been included here as they are generally considered to be self-prescribed recreational activities as opposed to specific clinical interventions.

## Equine-assisted therapy/therapeutic riding

*Description*

Therapeutic riding involves the provision of horse-riding lessons for people who are disabled or less mobile than others, under the supervision of a specially trained physiotherapist. The physiotherapist undertakes an initial assessment of the rider, including manual handling requirements, facilitates the planning of the riding programme and may work with the rider during lessons. The physiotherapist then works closely with the riding instructor to ensure that the therapy is appropriate for the individual's capabilities. Recreational riding is offered by the Riding for the Disabled Association, both for riders who will never be able to ride independently and for those who intend to train for international equestrian events for the disabled. While not a designated therapy *per se*, the experience enables riders to develop balance, muscle strength and confidence often giving them a dramatic new perspective on life and the world, particularly for wheelchair users.

Evidence: Therapeutic riding has been shown to assist in the development of muscular strength, coordination and balance and to encourage self confidence.

Safety: No evidence was found on therapeutic riding as a clinical modality or regarding its relative safety. Conversely, no evidence was found on any specific contraindications. Clients should be supervised at all times by professional physiotherapists and riding instructors.

## Bibliography

Candler C 2003 Sensory integration and therapeutic riding at Summer Camp: an occupational performance outcomes. Physical Occupational Therapy Pediatrics 23(3):51–64

Daly M 2000 Rehabilitation in the therapeutic riding arena. Rehabilitation Nurse 25(5):167–168

Hammer A, Nilsagard Y, Forsberg A et al 2005 Evaluation of therapeutic riding (Sweden) hippotherapy (United States). A single-subject experimental design study replicated in eleven patients with multiple sclerosis. Physiotherapy Theory and Practice 21(1):51–77

Land G, Errington-Povalac E, Paul S 2002 The effects of therapeutic riding on sitting posture in individuals with disabilities. Journal of Chronic Fatigue Syndrome 10(1):1–12

Liptak G S 2005 Complementary and alternative therapies for cerebral palsy. Mental Retardation and Developmental Disabilities Research Reviews 11(2):156–163

Snider L, Korner-Bitensky N, Kammenn C et al 2007 Horseback riding as therapy for children with cerebral palsy: is there evidence of its effectiveness? Physical Occupational Therapy Pediatrics 27(2):5–23

Winchester P, Kendall K, Peters H et al 2002 The effect of therapeutic horseback riding on gross motor function and gait speed in children who are developmentally delayed. Physical Occupational Therapy Pediatrics 22(3–4): 37–50

## Resources

Riding for the Disabled: www.riding-for-disabled.org.uk

## Hippotherapy

*Description*

Hippotherapy differs from therapeutic riding in that it is a specific physiotherapy treatment on horseback, for adults and children with varying degrees of physical, cognitive or emotional disability. The person sits passively on the horse's back without the conventional saddle, allowing for three-dimensional movement of the horse, thus helping to elicit automatic reactions from the rider as they accommodate to the horse's gait. The physiotherapist applies neurodevelopmental and sensory integration techniques to develop balance and posture, which programmes or re-programmes the mind via a feedback loop, allowing more normal movement to be developed. It also engenders self confidence, flexibility and muscle strength. When the person is unable to accommodate to the horse's movement, back riding is used in which a physiotherapist qualified in neurodevelopment and riding sits on the horse behind the person and facilitates techniques to encourage postural control. It is a labour-intensive therapy involving the therapist, a riding master who controls the horse and a side helper and is, consequently, expensive.

Evidence: Hippotherapy has been shown to develop muscular strength, coordination and balance and encourage self confidence.

Safety: No evidence was found regarding safety or specific contraindications.

### Bibliography

Benda W, McGibbon N, Grant K 2003 Improvements in muscle symmetry in children with cerebral palsy after equine assisted therapy (hippotherapy). Journal of Alternative Complementary Medicine 9(6):817–825

Gehrts K 2006 Examining the effectiveness of hippotherapy with cerebral palsy (Part 3). NZ Physiotherapy Krankengymnastik 59(10):1086–1093

Hammer A, Nilsagard Y, Forsberg A et al 2005 Evaluation of therapeutic riding (Sweden) hippotherapy (United States). A single-subject experimental design study replicated in eleven patients with multiple sclerosis. Physiotherapy Theory and Practice 21(1):51–77

Sterba J 2007 Does horseback riding or therapist-directed hippotherapy rehabilitate children with cerebral palsy? Developments Medical Child Neurology 49(1):68–73

### Resources

Chartered Society of Physiotherapists: www.csp.org.uk
Riding for the Disabled: www.riding-for-disabled.org.uk

## Pet therapy

### Description

Pet therapy was originally endorsed by Florence Nightingale who observed that pets were often excellent companions for the sick. It has since developed into a widely used therapy involving a range of interventions including: facilitating animals to visit people in hospital or convalescent homes, especially those who are away from home for long periods of time, the use of pets as part of a therapy programme and the training of dogs to facilitate independence in people who are disabled.

Evidence:   Stroking, watching or interacting with animals has been shown to reduce blood pressure, reduce anxiety and promote interaction and communication and elevate mood.

Safety:   Careful choice of animal is needed, caution with people who are allergic to animal dander or who are animal phobic or immunosuppressed.

### Bibliography

Malesle M 2004 Hospice care. Pet therapy. Hospice Health Network 78(11):24

Roenke L, Mulligan S 1998 The therapeutic value of the human-animal connection. Occupational Therapy Healthcare 11(2):27–43

### Resources

Pet Therapy: www.petsastherapy.org

## Anthroposophical medicine

*Description*

Anthroposophical medicine was developed by the Austrian philosopher, Rudolph Steiner, the name derived from the Greek anthropos (human) and sophia (wisdom). It is based on the concept of body, mind and spirit/ego and encompasses the life-force/etheric body and the soul/astral body. Health equates to maintenance of equilibrium between the four parts, in conjunction with earth, water, fire and air and is dependent on the balance between catabolism (breakdown and use of energy) and anabolism (building and storing of energy). Anthroposophical medicine also recognizes three interconnected dynamic systems: the nervous system (spinal column, brain and nerves, responsible for thought and cognition), metabolic system (responsible for assimilation of nutrition, metabolism and movement of the limbs) and the rhythmic system (responsible for respiratory and circulatory systems, i.e. the rhythms of the body). The nervous and metabolic systems are polar opposites, while the rhythmic system maintains the balance between the two. Illness is viewed as a transformation, as part of the person's destiny; failure to acknowledge this results in interference with the body/soul connection.

Anthroposophical medicine is normally practised by specially trained doctors and nurses and advocates a biodynamic, lacto-vegetarian diet, with unrefined carbohydrates. Foods are analogous with the human body; plant roots equate to the brain; stems/leaves equate to the rhythmic system; flowers/fruit equate to the metabolic system. Massage, hydrotherapy, eurhythmy, art, music therapy, homeopathic and herbal remedies are used as well as some conventional interventions. Consideration is given to seasonal and cosmic influences, i.e. solar, lunar and planetary influences, with treatments prescribed both for physical effects and as a catalyst in promoting the person's life-force.

Evidence: There appears to be no real scientific evidence for anthroposophical medicine as a concept, although individual aspects have been evaluated. It is therefore necessary to have a basic knowledge of the elements of the therapy in order to conduct professional literature searches on both its effectiveness and safety. Therapeutic eurythmy may be useful for children with attention deficit hyperactivity disorder (ADHD). Herbal remedies used in anthroposophical medicine, such as Iscador (mistletoe) have been found to regulate cardiorespiratory function during night-time sleep and may prolong survival time in oncology patients.

Safety:  As this is an integrated medical system safety issues relate to the individual components and the professional accountability of the practitioners.

Bibliography

Arman M, Backman M 2000 A longitudinal study on women's experiences of life with breast cancer in anthroposophical (complementary) and conventional care. European Journal of Cancer Care 16(5):440–450

Cysarz D, Heckmann C, Bettermann H et al 2002 Effects of an anthroposophical remedy on cardiorespiratory regulation. Alternative Therapies in Health and Medicine 8(6):78–83

Ernst E 2004 Anthroposophical medicine: a systematic review of randomised clinical trials. Wiener klinische Wochenschrift 116(4):128–130

Fliostrup H, Swartz J, Bergstgrom A et al 2006 Allergic disease and sensitization in Steiner school children. Journal of Allergy and Clinical Immunology 117(1):59–66

Grossarth-Maticek R, Kiene H, Baumgartner S M et al 2001 Use of Iscador, an extract of European mistletoe (Viscum album), in cancer treatment: prospective nonrandomized and randomized matched-pair studies nested within a cohort study. Alternative Therapies in Health and Medicine 7(3):57–66, 68–72

Hamre H, Becker-Witt C, Glockman A et al 2004 Anthroposophical therapies in chronic disease: the Anthroposophical Medicine Outcomes Study (AMOS). European Journal of Medical Research 9(7):351–360

Hamre H, Fischer M, Heger M et al 2005 Anthroposophical vs. conventional therapy of acute respiratory and ear infections: a prospective outcomes study. Wiener klinische Wochenschrift 117(7–8):256–268

Heusser P, Berger-Brauna S, Ziegler R 2006 Palliative in-patient cancer treatment in an anthroposophical hospital: 1. Treatment patterns and compliance with anthroposophical medicine. Forschende Komplementärmedizin und Klassische Naturheilkunde 13(2):94–100

Majorek M, Tüchelmann T, Heusser P 2004 Therapeutic eurhythmy-movement therapy for children with attention deficit hyperactivity disorder (ADHD): a pilot study. Complementary Therapies in Nursing and Midwifery 10(1):46–53

Van der Bie G and Huber M 2003 Foundations of Anthroposophical Medicine: A Training Manual. Floris Books, Edinburgh

---

### Resources

Anthroposophy Organization: www.anthroposophy.org
Weleda: www.weleda.co.uk

## Aromatherapy

*Description*

Aromatherapy is the therapeutic use of concentrated essential oils administered via the skin in massage, creams, gels and in water, via the respiratory tract in inhalations and vaporizers via mucous membranes, including rectally and vaginally, plus, occasionally gastrointestinally (aromatology). Therapeutic effects are thought to result from a combination of the chemical constituents, methods of administration and the effects of the aromas. The French chemist, Rene-Maurice Gattefosse (1881–1950) first used the term 'aromatherapie' and promoted essential oils as medical interventions after he burnt his hand in an accident and found that lavender oil relieved the pain and aided healing. The French surgeon Dr Jean Valnet (1920–1975) subsequently used essential oils effectively to treat wounded soldiers during the First World War and continued his research, teaching and practice almost until his death.

Essential oils are extracted most commonly by steam distillation, although other methods such as expression (for citrus essences) and solvent extraction (which produces an absolute) are also used. They contain hundreds of constituents with different therapeutic properties, grouped primarily into: alcohols (antiseptic, antiviral), aldehydes (antiseptic, sedative), coumarins (anticoagulant, hypotensive, phototoxic), esters (antifungal, antispasmodic, sedative), ketones (expectorant, mucolytic, analgesic, possibly emmenagogic), oxides (expectorant), terpenes – sub-divided into monoterpenes (antibacterial antiviral, analgesic), sesquiterpenes (antiinfective, antiinflammatory, antispasmodic) and diterpenes (antiinfective, expectorant), as well as phenols (antibacterial, stimulants) and some other constituents.

## Evidence

There is both clinical and non-clinical evidence that essential oils are antibacterial, antiviral and antifungal and trials have demonstrated their effectiveness in combating methicillin resistant staphylococcus aureus (MRSA) and other major infections. Clinical studies have demonstrated the value of aromatherapy for labour and other types of pain, reducing blood pressure, anxiety, depression and insomnia but whether this is due to the essential oil chemistry or the method of administration has not yet been adequately verified. Many of the aromatherapy trials have investigated the concept of aromatherapy as a treatment modality, irrespective of the individual oils used. The number of studies on specific essential oils varies, with some, such as tea tree, having vast amounts of evidence, while others which are less well known or less commonly used, have very little, if any, literature to support them. References to clinical research, as well as some case reports, have been included here, where available; readers interested in non-clinical investigations of specific oils are referred to the *Journal of Essential Oil Research* as one particularly good resource.

Safety: Essential oils should be stored in dark bottles at a cool temperature, to avoid deterioration and be kept away from children. Some oils such as citrus oils will deteriorate more quickly than others and have a shelf-life of about 3–6 months; they should be stored in the refrigerator. In the UK, oils are not normally ingested as it is not possible to determine the site and rate of absorption, nor can the majority of UK aromatherapists obtain indemnity insurance cover for administration by mouth (although French doctors prescribe oils orally). Oils should not normally be applied neat to the skin, as dermal sensitivity may occur, but should be diluted in a carrier oil, such as grapeseed or sweet almond (although some individuals may also be sensitive to certain carrier oils, particularly sweet almond). Blended oils should be discarded after about 4 weeks as oxidation (deterioration) may chemically alter the oil and its therapeutic properties.

Some oils should be avoided by people with abnormalities of blood pressure, as certain essential oils are hypotensive, while others are hypertensive. If used in large doses, certain oils, notably the citrus oils, may cause photosensitivity in susceptible people and in those taking drugs with similar side-effects. There are many essential oils which should not be used by pregnant or lactating women, as the effects on the fetus and the mother's systemic condition are unknown; it is advisable to avoid all essential oils in pregnancy unless recommended by a suitably trained practitioner. Many oils should be used with caution in small children under 12 years of age and should never be used on babies under 3 months, as the antibacterial properties may adversely affect ongoing maturation of the immune system.

Dosages should range from 0.5–1% for children; 1–2% during pregnancy, labour and lactation and for patients compromised by illness or debilitating conditions; the normal dose for healthy adults is up to 3% ( a total of 3 drops of essential oil in each 5 mL of carrier/base oil). Care should be taken if the individual is prescribed any medication since the metabolism of essential oils is precisely the same as for pharmacological drugs and there is a theoretical possibility of drug–oil interactions.

## Bibliography

Bastard J, Tiran D 2006 Aromatherapy and massage for antenatal anxiety: its effect on the fetus. Complementary Therapies in Clinical Practice 12(1): 48–54

Burns E, Zobbi V, Panzeri D et al 2007 Aromatherapy in childbirth: a pilot randomised controlled trial. British Journal of Obstetrics and Gynaecology 114(7):838–844

Hadfield N 2001 The role of aromatherapy massage in reducing anxiety in patients with malignant brain tumours. International Journal of Palliative Nursing 7(6):279–285

Hur M H, Oh H, Lee M S et al 2007 Effects of aromatherapy massage on blood pressure and lipid profile in Korean climacteric women. International Journal of Neuroscience 117(9):1281–1287

Fellowes D, Barnes K, Wilkinson S 2004 Aromatherapy and massage for symptom relief in patients with cancer. Cochrane Database of Systematic Reviews(2), CD002287

Kim J T, Ren C J, Fielding G A et al 2007 Treatment with lavender aromatherapy in the post-anesthesia care unit reduces opioid requirements of morbidly obese patients undergoing laparoscopic adjustable gastric banding. Obstetric Surgery 17(7):920–925

Kyle G 2006 Evaluating the effectiveness of aromatherapy in reducing levels of anxiety in palliative care patients: results of a pilot study. Complementary Therapies in Clinical Practice 12(2):148–155

Lee C O 2003 Clinical aromatherapy Part II: Safe guidelines for integration into clinical practice. Clinical Journal of Oncology Nursing 7(5):597–598

Lin P W, Chan W C, Ng B F et al 2007 Efficacy of aromatherapy (Lavandula angustifolia) as an intervention for agitated behaviours in Chinese older persons with dementia: a cross-over randomized trial. International Journal of Geriatric Psychiatry 22(5):405–410

Lis-Balchin M 1999 Possible health and safety problems in the use of novel plant essential oils and extracts in aromatherapy. Journal of the Royal Society of Health 4:240–243

Lis-Balchin M 2006 Aromatherapy Science: A Guide for Healthcare Professionals. Pharmaceutical Press, London

Tiran D 2004 Clinical Aromatherapy for Pregnancy and Childbirth, 2nd edn. Churchill Livingstone, Edinburgh

Wilkinson S M, Love S B, Westcombe A M et al 2007 Effectiveness of aromatherapy massage in the management of anxiety and depression in patients with cancer: a multicenter randomized controlled trial. Journal of Clinical Oncology 25(5):532–539

Resources

Aromatherapy Organisations Council: http://www.aocuk.net

# Selected essential oils

*Basil* (Ocimum basilicum)

Traditional uses:    antibacterial, antifungal, stimulant, expectorant.

Principal constituents: linalool, 1, 8 cineol, eugenol, pinene, camphor, methyl chavicol, β-caryophyllene.

Evidence:    There is some evidence of the antiinfective properties of basil oil.

Safety:    Mildly toxic, not for oral administration, has previously been thought to be carcinogenic. Not to be used in pregnancy or for children.

Bibliography

Misner B D 2007 A novel aromatic oil compound inhibits microbial overgrowth on feet: a case study. Journal of the International Society of Sports Nutrition 4:3

*Benzoin* (Styrax benzoin)

Traditional uses:    respiratory tract infection, skin lesions, warming and soothing.

Principal constituents:    benzoic acid, vanillin, aldehydes.

Evidence:    No evidence of therapeutic properties was found, although there are case reports on the potential adverse dermal effects.

Safety:    May cause dermal irritation. Not for oral administration. Appears safe in therapeutic doses.

Bibliography

Scardamaglia L, Nixon R, Fewings J 2003 Compound tincture of benzoin: a common contact allergen? Australasian Journal of Dermatology 44(3):180–184

*Bergamot* (Citrus bergamia)

Traditional uses:    urinary and respiratory tract infections, antimicrobial, mood enhancer.

Principal constituents:    linalyl acetate, limonene and linalool α- and β-terpinene.

Evidence: Most studies have focused on the antibacterial and antimicrobial effects of a number of essential oils, including bergamot. Safety: Non-toxic in therapeutic dosages, not for oral administration. May increase photosensitivity in susceptible people: avoid direct sunlight/sunbed use for at least 2h after administration May also cause dermal irritation. Safe in pregnancy and for children over 12 months. Shelf-life of 3–6 months when stored in refrigerator.

#### Bibliography

Fisher K, Phillips C A 2006 The effect of lemon orange and bergamot essential oils and their components on the survival of Campylobacter jejuni, Escherichia coli O157, Listeria monocytogenes, Bacillus cereus and Staphylococcus aureus in vitro and in food systems. Journal of Applied Microbiology 101(6):1232–1240

Kejlová K, Jírová D, Bendová H et al 2007 Phototoxicity of bergamot oil assessed by in vitro techniques in combination with human patch tests. Toxicology in Vitro 21(7):1298–1303

Sanguinetti M, Posteraro B, Romano L et al 2007 In vitro activity of Citrus bergamia (bergamot) oil against clinical isolates of dermatophytes. Journal of Antimicrobial Chemotherapy 59(2):305–308

## Black pepper (Piper nigrum)

Traditional uses: digestive disorders, antispasmodic, tonic, stimulant, warming.

Principal constituents: piperine, pinene, limonene, terpinolene, caryophyllene, cadinene.

Evidence: Single studies have demonstrated a possible role in smoking cessation and in its stimulating effect on the olfactory system. Safety: Safe in pregnancy and labour in low doses, not safe for children. Best avoided in those who are hyper-pyrexial, due to its warming properties.

#### Bibliography

Ebihara T, Ebihara S, Maruyama M et al 2006 A randomized trial of olfactory stimulation using black pepper oil in older people with swallowing dysfunction. Journal of the American Geriatrics Society 54(9):1401–1406

Rose J E, Behm F M 1994 Inhalation of vapor from black pepper extract reduces smoking withdrawal symptoms. Drug and Alcohol Dependence 34(3):225–229

*Cedarwood* (Cedrus atlanticus)

Traditional uses:   insect repellent, antiseptic, bronchial and urinary tract infections, catarrhal.

Principal constituents:   cedrol, cadinene sesquiterpenes terpenic hydrocarbons.

Evidence:   No specific evidence found.

Safety:   Safe in therapeutic dosages for healthy people. Probably not safe in pregnancy, but appears relatively safe for children over 6 months. Not for oral administration.

---

**Bibliography**

Hay I C, Jamieson Mormerod A D 1998 Randomized trial of aromatherapy Successful treatment for alopecia areata. Archives of Dermatology 134: 1349–1352

*Chamomile – Roman* (Anthemis nobilis)/*German/Hungarian* (Matricaria recutita)/*Moroccan* (Principal)

Traditional uses: antispasmodic, antiinflammatory, antiseptic, sedative, wound healing.

Principal constituents: coumarins, esters, terpenes, alcohol and ketone; chamazulene, which is formed during the extraction process and causes the oil to turn blue. Roman chamomile has high percentage of esters (antiinflammatory, antispasmodic, antifungal, calming and sedative); German chamomile oil contains more antiinflammatory chamazulene, produced when the essential oil is extracted from the plant. (Constituents vary between varieties.)

Evidence:   Any evidence should be set in context since most studies and case reports relate to effects of the whole plant, rather than just the extracted essential oil. However, experiential evidence suggests that chamomile has a sedating effect.

Safety:   Exceeding the recommended amount can result in a stimulating rather than sedating effect. May interact with warfarin if used in large doses. Roman chamomile should not be used in pregnancy until the third trimester due to higher proportion of camphor.

Bibliography

Segal R, Pilote L 2006 Warfarin interaction with Matricaria chamomilla. Canadian Medical Association Journal 174:1281–1282

Melzer J, Rosch W, Reichling J et al 2004 Meta-analysis: phytotherapy of functional dyspepsia with the herbal drug preparation STW 5 (Iberogast). Alimentary Pharmacology and Therapeutics 20:1279–1287

Nayak B S, Raju S S, Rao A V 2007 Wound healing activity of Matricaria recutita L – extract. Journal of Wound Care 16(7):298–302

Storr M, Sibaev A, Weiser D et al 2004 Herbal extracts modulate the amplitude and frequency of slow waves in circular smooth muscle of mouse small intestine. Digestion 70:257–264

## *Cinnamon* (Cinnamomum zeylanicum)

Traditional uses:   respiratory tract infections.

Principal constituents:   α-pinene, cinnamaldehyde, eugenol, caryophyllene.

Evidence:   May possibly have an anti-diabetic effect.

Safety:   Non-toxic in therapeutic dosages. Not for oral administration. May cause dermal irritation in susceptible people, in the form of contact dermatitis. Probably not safe during pregnancy, but appears safe for children over 6 months.

Bibliography

Kanerva L, Estlander T, Jolanki R 1996 Occupational allergic contact dermatitis from spices. Contact Dermatitis 35:157–162

Verspohl E J, Bauer K, Neddermann E 2005 Antidiabetic effect of Cinnamomum cassia and Cinnamomum zeylanicum in vivo and in vitro. Phytotherapy Research 19:203–206

## *Clary sage* (Salvia sclarea)

Traditional uses:   euphoric, antispasmodic, muscle relaxant, childbirth.

Principal constituents:   linalyl acetate, sclareol, linalool, salvene caryophyllene, composition may vary.

Evidence:   Although no studies have been undertaken specifically on clary sage in isolation, there does appear to be the suggestion that this essential oil has an effect on smooth muscle, such as the uterus.

Safety:   Non-toxic in therapeutic dosages when used appropriately. Not for oral administration. May potentiate the effects of alcohol. Completely contraindicated in pregnancy; may enhance uterine action in labour, but advise women not to use it to initiate uterine contractions towards term unless on the advice of a midwife. May cause menorrhagia and even inter-menstrual bleeding – caution with clients and therapists who are menstruating heavily. May cause transient hypotension.

### Bibliography

Burns E, Blamey C, Ersser S J et al 2000 The use of aromatherapy in intrapartum midwifery practice an observational study. Complementary Therapies in Nursing and Midwifery 6(1):33–34

Han S H, Hur M H, Buckle J et al 2006 Effect of aromatherapy on symptoms of dysmenorrhea in college students: a randomized placebo-controlled clinical trial. Journal of Alternative and Complementary Medicine 12(6):535–541

Lis-Balchin M, Hart S 1997 A preliminary study of the effect of essential oils on skeletal and smooth muscle in vitro. Journal of Ethnopharmacology 58(3):183–187

### *Cypress* (Cupressus sempervirens)

Traditional uses:    astringent, antispasmodic, for asthma, oedema, may aid weight loss, stimulating.

Principal constituents:    D-pinene, D-camphene, cymene, sabinol, camphor.

Evidence:    Appears to be effective in reducing fluid retention.

Safety:    Non-toxic in therapeutic dosages, safe in pregnancy and for children, not for oral administration, may cause dermal irritation.

### Bibliography

Kim H J 2007 Effect of aromatherapy massage on abdominal fat and body image in post-menopausal women. Taehan Kanho Hakhoe Chi 37(4):603–612

Lim W C, Seo J M, Lee C I et al 2005 Stimulative and sedative effects of essential oils upon inhalation in mice. Archives of Pharmacal Research 28(7):770–774

### *Eucalyptus* (Eucalyptus globules, E. radiate, E. citriodora)

Traditional uses: decongestant, mucolytic, antibacterial, local analgesic, CNS stimulant, deodorizing.

Principal constituents:    (may vary between genera) eucalyptol, ethyl alcohol, amyl alcohol aldehydes, camphene, pinene, menthone.

Evidence:    Shown to have strong antiinfective properties; also an effective expectorant.

Safety:    Not for oral use. Appears safe in pregnancy and for children over the age of 6 months, in therapeutic doses.

### Bibliography

Liapi C, Anifantis G, Chinou I et al 2007 Antinociceptive properties of 1,8-cineole and beta-pinene, from the essential oil of Eucalyptus camaldulensis leaves, in rodents. Planta Medica 73(12):1247–1254

Sartorelli P, Marquioreto A D, Amaral-Baroli A et al 2007 Chemical composition and antimicrobial activity of the essential oils from two species of Eucalyptus. Phytotherapy Research 21(3):231–233

Silva J, Abebe W, Sousa S M et al 2003 Analgesic and antiinflammatory effects of essential oils of eucalyptus. Journal of Ethnopharmacology 89:277–283

Warnke P H, Sherry E, Russo P A et al 2006 Antibacterial essential oils in malodorous cancer patients: clinical observations in 30 patients. Phytomedicine 13(7):463–467

## *Frankincense* (Boswellia carteri)

Traditional uses:    respiratory tract infections, asthma, urinary tract infections, used to calm and relax, aid to meditation, antiinflammatory, used for diarrhoea.

Principal constituents:    α-pinene, α-thujene, dipentene, cymene, farnesol, borneol, olibanol, limonene, linalool (may differ between oils from different locations).

Evidence:    Any evidence suggesting either an antiinfective analgesic effect is from studies in which several essential oils have been used in combination, thus it is difficult to ascertain whether the effects are specifically related to frankincense; experiential evidence seems to reflect the calming and pain-relieving properties with which frankincense has long been credited. It also appears to have a good expectorant effect and has been used in some commercial preparations for this purpose.

Safety:    Safe in pregnancy and in children over the age of 6 months. Not for oral use.

### Bibliography

Borrelli F, Capasso F, Capasso R et al 2006 Effect of Boswellia serrata on intestinal motility in rodents: inhibition of diarrhoea without constipation. British Journal of Pharmacology(4):553–560

Buckle J 1999 Use of aromatherapy as a complementary treatment for chronic pain. Alternative Therapies in Health and Medicine 5:42–51

Clarke J O, Mullin G E 2008 A review of complementary and alternative approaches to immunomodulation. Nutrition in Clinical Practice 23(1):49–62

## Geranium (Pelargonium graveolens)

Traditional uses: antidepressant, antiseptic, astringent, used for menopausal problems, antibacterial, antimicrobial, antiinflammatory. Principal constituents: citronellol, geraniol, linalool, citral, geranyl acetate, valerianic acid.

Evidence: Several reputable studies reflect the antibacterial and antimicrobial effects of geranium oil.

Safety: Non-toxic in normal doses, not for oral ingestion. Safe in pregnancy. May cause dermal irritation.

### Bibliography

Maruyama N, Ishibashi H, Hu W et al 2006 Suppression of carrageenan- and collagen II-induced inflammation in mice by geranium oil. Mediators of Inflammation 2006(3):62537

Prabuseenivasan S, Jayakumar M, Ignacimuthu S 2006 In vitro antibacterial activity of some plant essential oils. BMC Complementary and Alternative Medicine 6:39

Rosato A, Vitali C, De Laurentis N et al 2007 Antibacterial effect of some essential oils administered alone or in combination with norfloxacin. Phytomedicine 14(11):727–732

Schelz Z, Molnar J, Hohmann J 2006 Antimicrobial and antiplasmid activities of essential oils. Fitoterapia 77(4):279–285

## Ginger (Zingiber officinalis)

Traditional uses: warming, antispasmodic, used for stomach cramps and diarrhoea, may enhance uterine action, antibacterial, antiviral, stimulating. Antiemetic, although most research has investigated the herbal remedy rather than the essential oil. Possible role in converting breech-presenting fetus to cephalic.

Principal constituents: zingiberene, camphene, limonene, d-phellandrene, 1,8-cineole, geranial, geraniol, curcumene, linalool, citrale.

Evidence: Numerous studies confirm the antibacterial effects of ginger. Any apparent evidence on the use of ginger oil as an antiemetic need to be put in context as the majority of research has been undertaken using ginger root as a herbal remedy, rather than the extracted essential oil.

A single study suggests that ginger has an effect on the smooth muscle of the uterus, possibly indicating a role in obstetrics.

Safety: Not to be used by those with coagulation disorders or on anticoagulant medication (including NSAIs). Not always appropriate as an antiemetic in pregnancy, may cause heart burn. Non-toxic, safe in therapeutic dosages, essential oil not for oral consumption.

### Bibliography

Calvert I 2005 Ginger: an essential oil for shortening labour? Practising Midwife 8(1):30–34

Koch C, Reichling J, Schneele J et al 2008 Inhibitory effect of essential oils against herpes simplex virus type 2. Phytomedicine 15(1–2):71–78

Lim W C, Seo J M, Lee C I et al 2005 Stimulative and sedative effects of essential oils upon inhalation in mice. Archives of Pharmacol Research 28(7):770–774

Norajit K, Laohakunjit N, Kerdchoechuen O 2007 Antibacterial effect of five Zingiberaceae essential oils. Molecules 12(8):2047–2060

Riyazi A, Hensel A, Bauer K et al 2007 The effect of the volatile oil from ginger rhizomes (Zingiber officinale), its fractions and isolated compounds on the 5-HT3 receptor complex and the serotoninergic system of the rat ileum. Planta Medica 73(4):355–362

Zhou H L, Deng Y M, Xie Q M 2006 The modulatory effects of the volatile oil of ginger on the cellular immune response in vitro and in vivo in mice. Journal of Ethnopharmacology 105(1–2):301–305

## Grapefruit (Citrus paradisi)

Traditional uses: diuretic, detoxifier, lymphatic stimulant for fluid retention, weight loss, cellulite, acne, antiseptic, antibacterial, analgesic.

Principal constituents: limonene, citral, geraniol, neral, cadinene and paradisol.

Evidence: Some trials on the antibacterial properties of essential oils have included grapefruit. It is possible that the effect of the aroma of grapefruit on the olfactory mechanism can be stimulating.

Safety: Non-toxic in therapeutic dosages. Safe for children; safe in pregnancy after the first trimester. Not for oral administration. May cause dermal irritation, may increase susceptibility to photosensitivity. Shelf-life of 3–6 months when stored in refrigerator.

Bibliography

Edwards-Jones V, Buck R, Shawcross S G et al 2004 The effect of essential oils on methicillin-resistant Staphylococcus aureus using a dressing model. Burns 30(8):772–777

Niijima A, Nagai K 2003 Effect of olfactory stimulation with flavor of grapefruit oil and lemon oil on the activity of sympathetic branch in the white adipose tissue of the epididymis. Experimental Biology and Medicine 228(10):1190–1192

Shen J, Niijima A, Tanida M et al 2007 Mechanism of changes induced in plasma glycerol by scent stimulation with grapefruit and lavender essential oils. Neuroscience Letters 416(3):241–246

## *Jasmine* (Jasminum officinalis)

Traditional uses: uterine tonic to relieve pain and strengthen contractions, antidepressant, aphrodisiac.

Principal constituents: benzyl benzoate, benzyl acetate, 1,8-cineole, methyl anthranilate, farnesene, cis-jasmone, indol, linalool and linalyl acetate.

Evidence: Several German studies have suggested the effects of a number of essential oils on human concentration, including jasmine.

Safety: Non-toxic in therapeutic dosages. Should be avoided during pregnancy but is acceptable in labour and the puerperium. Safe for children over 6 months. Not for oral administration.

Bibliography

Imberger J, Heuberger E, Mahrhofer C et al 2001 The influence of essential oils on human attention and alertness. Chemical Senses 26(3):239–245

Lis-Balchin M, Hart S, Wan Hang Lo B 2002 Jasmine absolute (Jasminum grandiflora L.) and its mode of action on guinea-pig ileum in vitro. Phytotherapy Research 16(5):437–439

## *Lavender* (Lavandula angustifolia/augustifolia/officinalis, *true lavender*)

Traditional uses: sedative, relaxant, antispasmodic, antibacterial, antimicrobial, anti-hypertensive, may reduce anxiety, analgesic, good for pain in labour, may aid wound healing.

Principal constituents: lavandulol, lavandulyl acetate, camphor, geranyl, geraniol, linalool, 1,8-cineole, limonene. (Vary between genera.)

Evidence: Lavender oil appears to have calming and analgesic properties, as well as reducing blood pressure and improving circulation.

Safety:    Non-toxic in therapeutic dosages. Safe for children over the age of 6 months. *Lavandula angustifolia* appears safe after the first trimester of pregnancy, caution with other varieties of lavender which may contain higher levels of potentially emmenagogic constituents. Oxidized lavender may cause dermal irritation. Continual use in pre-pubertal boys have been shown to cause gynaecomastia. Not for oral administration.

Bibliography

Burns E, Blamey C, Ersser S J et al 2000 The use of aromatherapy in intrapartum midwifery practice: an observational study. Complementary Therapies in Nursing and Midwifery 6(1):33–34

Cline M, Taylor J E, Flores J et al 2008 Investigation of the anxiolytic effects of linalool, a lavender extract, in the male Sprague-Dawley rat. Arthroscopy Association of North America Journal 76(1):47–52

Hay I C, Jamieson M, Ormerod A D 1998 Randomized trial of aromatherapy: successful treatment for alopecia areata. Archives of Dermatology 134:1349–1352

Kim J T, Ren C J, Fielding G A et al 2007 Treatment with lavender aromatherapy in the post-anesthesia care unit reduces opioid requirements of morbidly obese patients undergoing laparoscopic adjustable gastric banding. Obesity Surgery 17(7):920–925

Kurtz J L 2007 Prepubertal gynecomastia linked to lavender and tea tree oils. New England Journal of Medicine 356(24):2542–2543

Shiina Y, Funabashi N, Lee K et al 2007 Relaxation effects of lavender aromatherapy improve coronary flow velocity reserve in healthy men evaluated by transthoracic Doppler echocardiography. International Journal of Cardiology 7, Aug [Epub ahead of print]

Sköld M, Hagvall L, Karlberg A T 2008 Autoxidation of linalyl acetate, the main component of lavender oil, creates potent contact allergens. Contact Dermatitis 58(1):9–14

Woollard A C, Tatham K C, Barker S 2007 The influence of essential oils on the process of wound healing: a review of the current evidence. Journal of Wound Care 16(6):255–257

## *Lemon* (Citrus limonum)

Traditional uses:    immunostimulant, antipyretic, circulatory stimulant, hypotensive.

Principal constituents:    citral, limonene, pinene, geraniol, neral, myrcene.

Evidence:    May be effective in reducing stress; studies on the antiinfective properties of essential oils in general have frequently included lemon oil.

Safety:   Non-toxic in therapeutic dosages. Safe for children over 6 months. Not for oral administration. Safe in pregnancy. May cause severe dermal irritation in susceptible people. Shelf-life of 3–6 months when stored in refrigerator.

### Bibliography

Fukumoto S, Sawasaki E, Okuyama S et al 2006 Flavor components of monoterpenes in citrus essential oils enhance the release of monoamines from rat brain slices. Nutritional Neuroscience 9(1–2):73–80

Komiya M, Takeuchi T, Harada E 2006 Lemon oil vapor causes an anti-stress effect via modulating the 5-HT and DA activities in mice. Behavioural Brain Research 172(2):240–249

### *Lemongrass* (Cymbopogon citrates)

Traditional uses:   antiseptic, antibacterial, analgesic for headaches.

Principal constituents:   citral, geraniol, farnesol, nerol, geraniol, citronellol, limonene and myrcene.

Evidence:   Appears to have antiinfective effects.

Safety:   Non-toxic in therapeutic dosages, safe for children over 6 months, not for oral administration, not recommended for massage in pregnancy.

### Bibliography

Duarte M C, Leme E E, Delarmelina C et al 2007 Activity of essential oils from Brazilian medicinal plants on Escherichia coli. Journal of Ethnopharmacology 111(2):197–201

Imura M, Misao H, Ushijima H 2006 The psychological effects of aromatherapy-massage in healthy postpartum mothers. Journal of Midwifery and Women's Health 51(2):e21–e27

Tampieri M P, Galuppi R, Macchioni F et al 2005 The inhibition of Candida albicans by selected essential oils and their major components. Mycopathologia 159(3):339–345

### *Marjoram sweet* (Origanum marjorana)

Traditional uses:  for respiratory tract infections, hypotensor, analgesic (headache, sciatica) intestinal problems constipation and diarrhoea and as a sedative.

Principal constituents:   1,8-cineole, linalool, limonene, carvacrol, thymol, terpinene, pinene, caryophyllene, geraniol, terpinolene.

Evidence: In common with many other essential oils, the majority of research has focused on the possible antiinfective properties of marjoram, particularly its antibacterial action.

Safety: Safe in therapeutic dosages, safe in pregnancy but caution in dermal application, may cause skin irritation, caution in children, not for oral administration.

### Bibliography

Kim M J, Nam E S, Paik S I 2005 The effects of aromatherapy on pain, depression and life satisfaction of arthritis patients. Taehan Kanho Hakhoe Chi 35(1):186–194

Oussalah M, Caillet S, Lacroix M 2006 Mechanism of action of Spanish oregano, Chinese cinnamon and savory essential oils against cell membranes and walls of Escherichia coli O157:H7 and Listeria monocytogenes. Journal of Food Protection 69(5):1046–1055

Ozcan M M, Sagdiç O, Ozkan G 2006 Inhibitory effects of spice essential oils on the growth of Bacillus species. Journal of Medicinal Food 9(3):418–421

## Neroli (Citrus aurantium)

Traditional uses: antidepressant, antispasmodic and sedative, antibacterial, antifungal; anti-hypertensive, premenstrual tension, menopausal symptoms, colic, diarrhoea.

Principal constituents: linalool, linalyl acetate, nerol, geraniol, citral, limonene.

Evidence: Very little contemporary evidence could be found. Older studies suggest a possible hypotensive effect; whether this is due to the chemical constituents or to the impact of the odour on the limbic system has not yet been satisfactorily demonstrated.

Safety: Safe in therapeutic dosages. May cause dermal irritation. Safe for children over 6 months. Safe in pregnancy.

### Bibliography

Campenni C E, Crawley E J, Meier M E 2004 Role of suggestion in odor-induced mood change. Psychological Reports 94(3 Pt 2):1127–1136

## Nutmeg (Myristica fragrans)

Traditional uses: warming and toning.

Principal constituents: camphene, myrcene, 1,8-cineole, terpinen-4-ol, sabinene, borneol, geraniol, linalool, eugenol, myristicin, safrole.

Evidence: Most available literature on evidence relates to the herbal medicine format of nutmeg, although it is the constituents of the volatile essential oils to which the adverse effects are attributed. However, much of the evidence concerns the oral consumption of nutmeg as a medicinal product, i.e. in amounts greater than the general culinary additive.

Safety: Not for oral administration. Can cause hallucinations, delirium, visual disturbances, ataxia and, ultimately, death. Potentially carcinogenic. Thought to be a cardiovascular stimulant. Totally contraindicated in pregnancy, although it may have a possible use, in extremely low doses, in labour. Contraindicated in children. Should not be used concurrently with morphine derivative drugs including codeine, pethidine, etc. May cause allergic dermatitis when applied to the skin.

Bibliography

Lis-Balchin M, Hart S 1997 A preliminary study of the effect of essential oils on skeletal and smooth muscle in vitro. Journal of Ethnopharmacology 58(3):183–187

Sangalli B C, Chiang W 2000 Toxicology of nutmeg abuse. Journal of Toxicology. Clinical Toxicology 38(6):671–678

*Orange (sweet)* (Citrus aurantium)

Traditional uses: antidepressant, antispasmodic, mild sedative, dyspepsia, colic, constipation.

Principal constituents: limonene, myrecene, pinene, sabanene, 1,8-cineole.

Evidence: May reduce anxiety, particularly when used in combination with other oils. Orange oil has been shown to have antiinfective effects, in similarity with other essential oils. Caution may be required when using this oil to combat traumatic effects, as the familiarity of the aroma and the impact of odour memory may trigger psychosomatic symptoms after the event.

Safety: Safe in therapeutic dosages. Safe for children over 6 months, safe in pregnancy, not for oral administration. Mildly irritant to skin. Avoid if sensitive to oranges. Shelf-life of 3–6 months when stored in a refrigerator.

Bibliography

Arias B A, Ramón-Laca L 2005 Pharmacological properties of citrus oils and their ancient and medieval uses in the Mediterranean region. Journal of Ethnopharmacology 97(1):89–95

Friedman M, Henika P R, Mandrell R E 2002 Bactericidal activities of plant essential oils and some of their isolated constituents against Campylobacter jejuni, Escherichia coli, Listeria monocytogenes and Salmonella enterica. Journal of Food Protection 65(10):1545–1560

Lehrner J, Marwinski G, Lehr S et al 2005 Ambient odors of orange and lavender reduce anxiety and improve mood in a dental office. Physiology and Behavior 86(1–2):92–95

## *Patchouli* (Pogostemon patchouli)

Traditional uses:   antiinflammatory, stimulant, tonic, antiseptic and febrifuge; used for depression, anxiety and stress-related conditions.

Principal constituents:   patchouline, eugenol, cadinene, α-guaiene, caryophyllene, pogostol, carvone; similar in structure to azulene found in chamomile.

Evidence:   May have antibacterial effects.

Safety:   Safe in therapeutic dosages, safe in pregnancy and children over 6 months, not for oral administration.

Bibliography

Edwards-Jones V, Buck R, Shawcross S G et al 2004 The effect of essential oils on methicillin-resistant Staphylococcus aureus using a dressing model. Burns 30(8):772–777

## *Peppermint* (Mentha piperata)

Traditional uses:   digestive problems, respiratory tract infections, antiemetic and for headaches and migraine.

Principal constituents:   menthol, limonene.

Evidence:   Peppermint is the only essential oil to be approved and included in the *British Pharmacopoeia* and has long been used for its carminative properties.

Safety:   Safe in therapeutic doses. Safe in pregnancy (but caution with dermal application). Safe in children over 6 months. Cardiac stimulant – caution in cardiac pathology. Skin irritant. Should not be used concurrently with homeopathic remedies as the strong aroma may inactivate the homeopathy.

## Bibliography

Forbes M A, Schmid M M 2006 Use of OTC essential oils to clear plantar warts. Nurse Practitioner 31(3), 53–55, 57

Hur M H, Park J, Maddock-Jennings W et al 2007 Reduction of mouth malodour and volatile sulphur compounds in intensive care patients using an essential oil mouthwash. Phytotherapy Research 21(7):641–643

Kim M A, Sakong J K, Kim E J et al 2005 Effect of aromatherapy massage for the relief of constipation in the elderly. Taehan Kanho Hakhoe Chi 35(1):56–64

Lim W C, Seo J M, Lee C I et al 2005 Stimulative and sedative effects of essential oils upon inhalation in mice. Archives of Pharmacol Research 28(7):770–774

Norrish M I, Dwyer K L 2005 Preliminary investigation of the effect of peppermint oil on an objective measure of daytime sleepiness. International Journal of Psychophysiology 55(3):291–298

Rafii F, Shahverdi A R 2007 Comparison of essential oils from three plants for enhancement of antimicrobial activity of nitrofurantoin against enterobacteria. Chemotherapy 53(1):21–25

## *Rose* (Rosa centifolia, Rosa damascene)

Traditional uses:   female disorders, useful in labour, antidepressant, particularly postnatal depression and generally for emotional imbalance, purported aphrodisiac.

Principal constituents:   citronellol, geraniol, nerol, linalool, phenylethyl alcohol. (Constituents may vary between species, some have high levels of ketones.)

Evidence:  Very little specific clinical research could be found, although general studies on the antibacterial effects of aromatherapy have often included rose oil.

Safety:  Safe in therapeutic dosages. Avoid until the latter part of pregnancy due to varying levels of ketones. Safe in children over 6 months. Not for oral administration. Ensure purity to avoid adulterated oils.

## Bibliography

Basim E, Basim H 2003 Antibacterial activity of Rosa damascena essential oil. Fitoterapia 74(4):394–396

Boskabady M H, Kiani S, Rakhshandah H 2006 Relaxant effects of Rosa damascena on guinea pig tracheal chains and its possible mechanism(s). Journal of Ethnopharmacology 106(3):377–382

Haze S, Sakai K, Gozu Y 2002 Effects of fragrance inhalation on sympathetic activity in normal adults. Japanese Journal of Pharmacology 90(3):247–253

## Rosemary (Rosmarinus officinalis)

Traditional uses:  antiseptic, CNS stimulant, useful for improving memory and concentration, for mental strain and exhaustion, an antispasmodic useful for dyspepsia, expectorant, used for respiratory infections and congestion, skin conditions such as seborrhoea and dandruff.

Principal constituents:  1,8-cineole, myrcene, pinene, limonene, borneol, linalool, ρ-cymene and camphor, camphene.

Evidence:  Appears to be strongly antibacterial. May have an impact on mood and concentration, particularly when inhaled.

Safety:  May cause epileptiform fits. Not for oral administration. Use with caution, in late pregnancy only. Not advised for children.

---

### Bibliography

Atsumi T, Tonosaki K 2007 Smelling lavender and rosemary increases free radical scavenging activity and decreases cortisol level in saliva. Psychiatry Research 150(1):89–96

Fu Y, Zu Y, Chen L et al 2007 Antimicrobial activity of clove and rosemary essential oils alone and in combination. Phytotherapy Research 21(10): 989–994

Gedney J J, Glover T L, Fillingim R B 2004 Sensory and affective pain discrimination after inhalation of essential oils. Psychosomatic Medicine 66(4):599–606

Luqman S, Dwivedi G R, Darokar M P et al 2007 Potential of rosemary oil to be used in drug-resistant infections. Alternative Therapies in Health and Medicine 13(5):54–59

Moss M, Cook J, Wesnes K et al 2003 Aromas of rosemary and lavender essential oils differentially affect cognition and mood in healthy adults. International Journal of Neuroscience 113(1):15–38

Prabuseenivasan S, Jayakumar M, Ignacimuthu S 2006 In vitro antibacterial activity of some plant essential oils. BMC Complementary and Alternative Medicine 6:39

## Rosewood (Aniba rosaeodora)

Traditional uses:  general tonic and relaxant, immunostimulant, analgesic, acne, colds and fever, urogenital conditions, fatigue.

Principal constituents:   linalool, α-terpineol, 1,8-cineole, nerol, geraniol.

Evidence:    No specific clinical research was found, although rosewood has been implicated, with other essential oils, in causing contact dermatitis.

Safety:    Safe in therapeutic dosages, safe in pregnancy, caution with children, not for oral administration, may cause dermal irritation.

### Bibliography

Schaller M, Korting H C 1995 Allergic airborne contact dermatitis from essential oils used in aromatherapy. Clinical and Experimental Dermatology 20(2):143–145

### *Sandalwood* (Santalum album)

Traditional uses: urinary tract infections, neuralgia, antiviral, antifungal, skin conditions, respiratory tract infections, decongestant and as a sedative.

Principal constituents: pinene, santalic acid, santalele farnesol, bisabolols, terasantalic acid.

Evidence:    Shown to have antiinfective properties. May also impact on mood and concentration.

Safety:    Safe in therapeutic dosages. Safe in pregnancy and for children over 6 months. Not for oral administration. Ensure the oil is ethically sourced where possible.

### Bibliography

Benencia F, Courrèges M C 1999 Antiviral activity of sandalwood oil against herpes simplex viruses-1 and -2. Phytomedicine 6(2):119–123

Heuberger E, Hongratanaworakit T, Buchbauer G 2006 East Indian Sandalwood and alpha-santalol odor increase physiological and self-rated arousal in humans. Planta Medica 72(9):792–800

Schnitzler P, Koch C, Reichling J 2007 Susceptibility of drug-resistant clinical herpes simplex virus type 1 strains to essential oils of ginger, thyme, hyssop and sandalwood. Antimicrobial Agents and Chemotherapy 51(5):1859–1862

### *Tea tree/ti tree* (Melaleuca alternifolia)

Traditional uses:    antibacterial, antiviral, antifungal, antimicrobial.

Principal constituents: $\alpha$-terpinene, pinene, limonene, sabinene, aromadendrene, terpinene, 1,8-cineole, y-terpene, p-cymene (terpinen-4-ol amounts may vary).

Evidence:    Several randomized controlled studies have demonstrated the effects of tea tree oil against specific pathogens, including Candidiasis (thrush), herpes and, more recently, against MRSA.

Safety:    Safe in therapeutic dosages. Safe in pregnancy but one study suggesting that tea tree may relax smooth muscle may mean it is best avoided in labour. Not safe for children due to high risk of skin irritation. May cause severe dermal irritation in susceptible people, caution in mucosal application (e.g. vaginal). Not for oral administration except diluted as a mouth wash. In common with lavender, prolonged use in boys has shown a risk of pre-pubertal gynaecomastia.

## Bibliography

Carson C F, Smith D W, Lampacher G J et al 2008 Use of deception to achieve double-blinding in a clinical trial of Melaleuca alternifolia (tea tree) oil for the treatment of recurrent herpes labialis. Contemporary Clinical Trials 29(1):9–12

Enshaieh S, Jooya A, Siadat A H et al 2007 The efficacy of 5% topical tea tree oil gel in mild to moderate acne vulgaris: a randomized, double-blind placebo-controlled study. Indian Journal of Dermatology, Venereology and Leprology 73(1):22–25

Henley D V, Lipson N, Korach K S et al 2007 Prepubertal gynecomastia linked to lavender and tea tree oils. New England Journal of Medicine 356(5): 479–485

Hur M H, Park J, Maddock-Jennings W et al 2007 Reduction of mouth malodour and volatile sulphur compounds in intensive care patients using an essential oil mouthwash. Phytotherapy Research 21(7):641–643

Kurtz J L 2007 Prepubertal gynecomastia linked to lavender and tea tree oils. New England Journal of Medicine 356(24):2542–2543

Mondello F, De Bernardis F, Girolamo A et al 2006 In vivo activity of terpinen-4-ol, the main bioactive component of Melaleuca alternifolia Cheel (tea tree) oil against azole-susceptible and -resistant human pathogenic Candida species. BMC Infectious Diseases 6:158

Park H, Jang C H, Cho Y B et al 2007 Antibacterial effect of tea-tree oil on methicillin-resistant Staphylococcus aureus biofilm formation of the tympanostomy tube: an in vitro study. In Vivo 21(6):1027–1030

Reichling J, Landvatter U, Wagner H et al 2006 In vitro studies on release and human skin permeation of Australian tea tree oil (TTO) from topical formulations. European Journal of Pharmaceutics and Biopharmaceutics 64(2):222–228

Rutherford T, Nixon R, Tam M et al 2007 Allergy to tea tree oil: retrospective review of 41 cases with positive patch tests over 4.5 years. Australasian Journal of Dermatology 48(2):83–87

Terzi V, Morcia C, Faccioli P et al 2007 In vitro antifungal activity of the tea tree (Melaleuca alternifolia) essential oil and its major components against plant pathogens. Letters in Applied Microbiology 44(6):613–618

Williams J D, Nixon R L, Lee A 2007 Recurrent allergic contact dermatitis due to allergen transfer by sunglasses. Contact Dermatitis 57(2):120–121

Woollard A C, Tatham K C, Barker S 2007 The influence of essential oils on the process of wound healing: a review of the current evidence. Journal of Wound Care 16(6):255–257

## *Thyme* (Thymus vulgaris)

Traditional uses:   as a digestive stimulant for gastric infections, colds and sore throats and respiratory tract infections.

Principal constituents:   thymol, carvacrol, geraniol, geranyl acetate, β-caryophyllene, α-pinene, ρ-cymene, 1,8-cineole, terpinolene.

Evidence:   Strongly antiinfective.

Safety:   Safe in therapeutic dosages. Avoid in pregnancy. Not safe for children. Not for oral administration. May cause dermal and mucous membrane irritation; may cause allergic reactions.

### Bibliography

Fabio A, Cermelli C, Fabio G et al 2007 Screening of the antibacterial effects of a variety of essential oils on microorganisms responsible for respiratory infections. Phytotherapy Research 21(4):374–377

Schnitzler P, Koch C, Reichling J 2007 Susceptibility of drug-resistant clinical herpes simplex virus type 1 strains to essential oils of ginger, thyme, hyssop and sandalwood. Antimicrobial Agents and Chemotherapy 51(5):1859–1862

Tullio V, Nostro A, Mandras N et al 2007 Antifungal activity of essential oils against filamentous fungi determined by broth microdilution and vapour contact methods. Journal of Applied Microbiology(6):1544–1550

## *Ylang ylang* (Cananga odorata)

Traditional uses:   antidepressant, anti-anxiety, soothing and sedative. May reduce blood pressure.

Principal constituents:   linalool, geraniol, farnesol, benzyl salicylate, eugenol, β-caryophyllene, methyl benzoate.

Evidence:   Studies appear to confirm the relaxation and calming effects of ylang ylang.

Safety: Safe in therapeutic dosages. Safe in pregnancy. Safe for children over 6 months. Not for oral administration. Check purity to avoid adulterated oil.

### Bibliography

Hongratanaworakit T, Buchbauer G 2006 Relaxing effect of ylang ylang oil on humans after transdermal absorption. Phytotherapy Research 20(9):758–763

Imberger J, Heuberger E, Mahrhofer C et al 2001 The influence of essential oils on human attention and alertness. Chemical Senses(3):239–245

## Bach flower remedies

*Description*

Flower remedies in general are forms of vibrational or energy medicine in which the essences distilled from various flowers are used to promote mental, emotional or physical healing. Flower remedies native to Great Britain include Bach flower remedies, the most well-known, as well as Bailey essences, Findhorn flower essences, Green man tree essences, Harebell remedies and Orchid flower essences. Other cultures have their own native systems, e.g. Australian bush flower essences, Alaskan flower essences, Californian research essences, Hawaiian flower essences, Pegasus essences, Himalayan aditi flower essences, Pacific essences. This book has not included the other systems of flower essences, since they are not as commonly used as Bach, at least not in the UK, but while the precise plants used differ in other systems, the principals are similar to those for Bach remedies.

Bach flower remedies were devised by Dr Edward Bach (1886–1936), a bacteriologist and homeopath, who abandoned conventional medicine to develop a more natural, gentle form of healing based on plants, prescribed to address emotional and spiritual health. There are 38 remedies, plus the Rescue Remedy. Liquid preparations (mother tinctures) are made from the petals of the relevant plants, combined with water ethanol mixtures. They are produced either by the sun method or by the boiling method. In the sun method, the flowering heads of the plants are placed in a bowl of pure spring water and left in the sun for 3 hours, after which time the water is preserved in brandy. For the boiling method, the relevant parts of the plant or tree are boiled in pure spring water for 30 min and left to cool; the water is then diluted in brandy. The remedies are clustered according to seven emotional states: fear, uncertainty, insufficient interest in the present, loneliness, oversensitivity, despondency/despair and over-concern for others. The 38 remedies and the Rescue Remedy are detailed below.

Diagnosis is achieved by the technique of 'peeling the onion' – finding out how a particular state of mind has been reached. For example, a state of insecurity may be caused by fear therefore the predominating emotion of fear would be diagnosed and treated. Treatment involves the selection of up to six remedies according to the individual's condition: 2 drops of each remedy are added to a 20 mL bottle of still spring water and the person is then instructed to use four drops of this at intervals prescribed by the practitioner. It is also possible to self-prescribe, relatively easily, although for more severe psychological states, individuals should be advised to consult a qualified practitioner.

Evidence:  The only studies undertaken appear to have been those on Rescue Remedy to relieve stress and anxiety, particularly pre-examination nerves, the efficacy of which has been largely attributed to the placebo effect. Flower remedies may have a part to play in the psycho-physiological aspects of pain control, but whether this is a placebo effect or not remains to be demonstrated. One particular study concluded that the remedies do not appear to be effective in helping children with attention deficit disorder.

Safety:  Mother tinctures, from which the individual essences are produced, contain alcohol, suggesting caution if the patient is a recovering alcoholic, taking specific drugs to assist alcohol dependence or metronidazole or who has a moral or religious objection to alcohol. There is no evidence of toxicity and remedies appear to be safe for children and during pregnancy, despite the recommendations to curb antenatal alcohol consumption. The tendency of the remedies to reveal underlying emotions, through the 'onion peeling' effect mean that the practitioner should possess adequate listening and counselling skills and be able to recognize when it is appropriate to stop treatment and refer to a specialist counsellor.

Bibliography

Ernst E 2002 'Flower remedies': a systematic review of the clinical evidence. Wiener klinische Wochenschrift 114(23–24):963–966

Howard J 2007 Do Bach flower remedies have a role to play in pain control? A critical analysis investigating therapeutic value beyond the placebo effect and the potential of Bach flower remedies as a psychological method of pain relief. Complementary Therapies in Clinical Practice 13(3):174–183

Pintov S, Hochman M, Livne A et al 2005 Bach flower remedies used for attention deficit hyperactivity disorder in children – a prospective double blind controlled study. European Journal of Paediatric Neurology 9(6):395–398

Walach H, Rilling C, Engelke U 2001 Efficacy of Bach-flower remedies in test anxiety: a double-blind, placebo-controlled, randomized trial with partial crossover. Journal of Anxiety Disorders 15(4):359–366

### Resources

Dr Edward Bach Centre, Wallingford, Oxon OX10 0PZ: www.bachcentre.com

## The 38 Bach flower remedies

Agrimony: for distress caused by hidden fears, worries and unhappiness.

Aspen: for fear of unknown origin.

Beech: for people who are intolerant and overcritical of others.

Centaury: to promote inner strength and re-balance those who are weak-willed or subservient, enabling them to stand up for themselves.

Cerato: to reduce indecision and promote confidence in own judgement.

Cherry plum: to reduce frightening thoughts and ideas, fear of loss of control and to promote clear rational thoughts.

Chestnut bud: for those who are unable to learn from past experience and constantly repeat the same mistakes.

Chicory: for over-possessiveness, manipulation and control of other people, particularly family; promotes a more balanced, undemanding love.

Clematis: to reduce day dreaming and absentmindedness and promote more awareness and sharpen focus on the 'here and now'.

Crab apple: is a cleansing remedy for those who feel their body or mind is somehow 'dirty' and has been contaminated, leading to obsessive thoughts or rituals.

Elm: for temporary lack of confidence and discouragement in normally confident and capable people.

Gentian: to dispel feelings of despondency and discouragement, usually resulting from disappointment.

Gorse: for feelings of hopelessness and despair, often for no reason.

Heather: to re-balance traits of self absorption and obsession with own illnesses or worries with a lack of awareness of other people or their needs leading to them being avoided and becoming lonely.

Holly: to counter feelings of jealousy, envy, spitefulness or suspicion.

Honeysuckle: for feelings of excessive homesickness, nostalgia, regrets, dwelling in the past.

Hornbeam: for lethargy, lack of enthusiasm, the 'Monday morning feeling'.

Impatiens: to help people who are quick in thought and action and whose desire for immediate results makes them impatient and quick tempered with others.

Larch: for lack of confidence and belief in own abilities.

Mimulus: to help the type of person who is very shy or nervous particularly to help a known fear or anxiety.

Mustard: to alleviate depression of unknown cause.

Oak: to help stoic committed individuals whose determination is undermined by overwork or illness and who refuse to seek help or rest, causing despondency or despair.

Olive: for tiredness and exhaustion due to either mental or physical overwork.

Pine: to counter feelings of guilt.

Red chestnut: for those who are over-concerned for the safety and well-being of others.

Rescue Remedy: a composite remedy consisting of Star of Bethlehem, Rock Rose, Impatiens, Cherry Plum and Clematis, used as a treatment for shock, panic and general reaction to emergencies or as part of a broader, composite remedy with other remedies. It is also available as a cream or spray.

Rock rose: used to combat feelings of terror and panic.

Rock water: for those who are rigid and self disciplined leading to narrowness of mind.

Scleranthus: to help those who are indecisive, mentally distressed at having to make even the smallest decision.

Star of Bethlehem: used as a remedy for severe shock.

Sweet chestnut:   to ease deep depression and despair caused by emotional pain.

Vervain:   to temper overenthusiasm for causes which leave the patient stressed, angry and frustrated.

Vine:   for the over-domineering, inflexible individual.

Walnut:   to facilitate change when adjustment is difficult; protects against external influences which might make choices or adjustments difficult.

Water violet:   to ease the isolation which can occur if people are too reserved, proud or aloof, resulting in them becoming cut off from enjoying the help or company of others.

White chestnut:   for mental arguments or unwanted thoughts which interfere with the person's peace of mind.

Wild oat:   to help people who are undecided in their path in life.

Wild rose:   for lack of motivation and apathy.

Willow:   for self pity, resentfulness and bitterness.

## Biochemic (biochemical) tissue salts

*Description*

This therapy was developed by William Schussler (1821–1898), a German physician, biochemist and homeopath. There are 12 biochemical tissue salts in the original range, used to re-balance and correct the body's own mineral salts, assumed to be essential to health at a cellular level. Deficiency of one or more of these mineral salts affects functioning of the others, leading to ill-health, but tissue salts can only be used to treat relative deficiencies, not absolute ones. Tissue salts are prepared according to homeopathic principles, using dynamized preparations in a low potency, usually 6× and are prescribed according to the presenting symptoms rather than being individualized to the person. They can be taken singly or in combination depending on the condition. Changes in diet and lifestyle may lead to the addition of new tissue salts to the original range in the near future, e.g. copper, manganese and zinc.

Evidence:    No clinical evidence for the use of these salts in the treatment of any specific condition could be found.

Safety:    No information regarding safety or evidence of specific contraindications was found.

Bibliography

No professional literature specifically on the complementary therapy concept of biochemic tissue salts could be found. Literature searches for the individual tissue salts identified research on the individual minerals, but not on the homeopathically prepared tissue salts.

## The tissue salts

Calcium fluoride:    builds elastic tissue of the body, muscles and blood vessels and is present in teeth and on bone surfaces. It is prescribed for: muscle weakness, dental decay, poor circulation, damaged muscles and bones, skin conditions and bleeding gums.

Calcium phosphate:    is present in bone and aids the formation of new blood vessels and digestion. It is prescribed for bone weakness, indigestion, poor circulation, fatigue and general debility and is thought to be good for convalescence.

Calcium sulphate:    purifies the blood and is an hepatic stimulant. It is prescribed for skin problems, mouth ulcers, slow healing wounds, neuralgia and catarrh.

Ferrum phosphate:    carries oxygen around the body and strengthens blood vessel walls. It is prescribed for respiratory problems, bleeding, anaemia, menorrhagia, throbbing headaches, pyrexia, inflammation, rheumatism. This tissue salt is often referred to as the 'first aid salt' when applied to wounds and is said to stem bleeding.

Kalium muriaticum:    is a blood conditioner prescribed for respiratory problems such as coughs, colds, bronchitis, swollen glands, childhood eczema and for digestive disorders.

Kalium phosphate:    is a nerve nutrient, present in brain cells and nerve tissue. It is used for physical and mental neurological system conditions, insomnia, mental and physical exhaustion, poor memory and concentration.

Kalium sulphate: oxygenates the tissues and cells of the body and is used for skin, hair and scalp and nail problems, as well as catarrh, hot flushes and chills.

Magnesium phosphate: is an antispasmodic which ensures smooth muscle movement and is prescribed for cramps, spasms, relief from sharp pains, flatulence, hiccups, headaches with shooting pains, low energy and neuralgia.

Natrum muriaticum: aids water metabolism, moisturizes the tissues and assists glandular function and digestion. It is used for dryness or excessive moisture in any part of the body, watery colds and sneezing, dry lips, dry itchy skin and eyes, hay fever, loss of taste or smell, headaches with constipation, thirst with craving for salty foods, sleep disturbance, fatigue and feelings of helplessness.

Natrum phosphate: neutralizes acid and aids assimilation of fatty acids. It helps to regulate hepatic and biliary function and is used for acidity, stomach upsets, heartburn, colic, indigestion, rheumatic pain and stiffness, swollen joints, jaundice and nausea.

Natrum sulphate: eliminates excess water and helps to maintain hepatic and biliary health. It is used for water retention, influenza, liver and gall bladder conditions, including jaundice, hepatitis, digestive upset, nausea and rheumatism.

Silica: is a cleanser and detoxifier, present in blood, skin, nails, hair bones and connective tissue. It is prescribed for spots, boils, styes, abscesses and other purulent skin conditions, cracked, brittle or split nails, glandular disorders, involuntary twitching of eyes or face muscles, stress and rheumatic pain.

## Bodywork therapies

*Description*

'Bodywork' is a generic term used to describe manual, postural and touch therapies which are part of the healing tradition of 'laying on of hands' and which subscribe to the basic tenets of symmetry, posture, coordinated movement and gravity, aiming towards bodily re-alignment, balance and efficient function. Some manual therapies, such as Chinese tuina and Japanese shiatsu, may also be referred to as energy medicine and are included in other relevant sections of this book.

## Alexander technique

*Description*

Alexander technique is a system of physical re-education to correct postural defects and habitual patterns of movement and bearing. It was devised by Frederick Alexander, an actor, who developed the system, following his own voice production problems, which he recognized as being due to defective posture and breathing associated with anxiety and 'stage nerves'. Treatment involves one-to-one lessons with practitioners who act as 'teachers' rather than therapists. Emphasis is on balance, breathing, posture, coordination and recognition of bodily tensions which have previously gone unnoticed and treatment aims to teach ways of moving, sitting, standing and walking to reduce strain on the bones, joints and muscles. It can be used occasionally to attend to acute problems, but is more generally viewed as a complete way of life which requires a degree of commitment from the individual.

Evidence: Some clinical trials indicate the value of the technique for coordination problems such as Parkinson's disease and for musculoskeletal problems, including those occurring during pregnancy.

Safety: No information regarding safety, contraindications and precautions was found.

Bibliography

Cacciatore T W, Horak F B, Henry S M 2005 Improvement in automatic postural coordination following Alexander technique lessons in a person with low back pain. Physical Therapy 85(6):565–578

Ernst E, Canter P H 2003 The Alexander technique: a systematic review of controlled clinical trials. Forschende Komplementärmedizin und Klassische Naturheilkunde 10(6):325–329

Jain S, Janssen K, DeCelle S 2004 Alexander technique and Feldenkrais method: a critical review. Physical Medicine and Rehabilitation Clinics of North America 15(4):811–825

Mehling W E, DiBlasi Z, Hecht F 2005 Bias control in trials of bodywork: a review of methodological issues. Journal of Alternative and Complementary Medicine 11(2):333–342

Schlinger M 2006 Feldenkrais method, Alexander technique and yoga – body awareness therapy in the performing arts. Physical Medicine and Rehabilitation Clinics of North America 17(4):865–875

Stallibrass C, Hampson M 2001 The Alexander technique: its application in midwifery and the results of preliminary research into Parkinson's. Complementary Therapies in Nursing and Midwifery 7(1):13–18

Stallibrass C, Frank C, Wentworth K 2005 Retention of skills learnt in Alexander technique lessons: 28 people with idiopathic Parkinson's disease. Journal of Bodywork and Movement Therapies 9:150–157

### Resources

Society of Teachers of the Alexander Technique: www.stat.org.uk

## Aston-patterning

*Description*

This is an integrative therapy of movement education (neurokinetics), ergonomics (identifying environmental aspects), bodywork (Aston massage, mykinetics, arthrokinetics) and fitness training (self massage, stretching, toning and cardiovascular fitness), based on the premise that all body movement consists of weight transfer, rocking across the hip and leg hinge joints, with matching flexion and extension of the spine, arms and legs. It incorporates reduction of the inherent tension of three-dimensional spiral patterns of movement and the aim is to develop a self awareness in order to achieve the required movement with minimal stress and maximum efficiency.

Evidence:  No evidence in the form of clinical trials or case reports on the efficacy of Aston-patterning could be found, although case reports on its use with children with cerebral palsy have previously been published.

Safety:  No information regarding safety, contraindications or precautions was found.

### Bibliography

Hannon J 2005 A review of Aston-patterning. Journal of Bodywork Movement Therapy 9(4):260–269

Liptak G S 2005 Complementary and alternative therapies for cerebral palsy. Mental Retardation and Developmental Disabilities Research Reviews 11(2): 156–163

## Bowen technique

*Description*

This is a very gentle technique developed by Tom Bowen (1916– 1982), an Australian healer in the 1950s. It is a manual therapy which incorporates a movement involving rolling of the fingers and thumb in order to manipulate soft tissues, thus stimulating energy flow and initiating self healing. The pressure applied by the fingers and thumb is no more than could be tolerated by applying pressure on an eyeball. Treatment sessions involve frequent breaks to facilitate the body to absorb the healing interventions from the therapist.

Evidence:   There is some evidence to suggest that this technique may help with musculoskeletal conditions including frozen shoulder.

Safety:   No specific information regarding safety, contraindications or precautions could be found in the literature.

### Bibliography

Carter B 2001 A pilot study to evaluate the effectiveness of Bowen technique in the management of clients with frozen shoulder. Complementary Therapies in Medicine 9(4):208–215

Carter B 2002 Clients' experiences of frozen shoulder and its treatment with Bowen technique. Complementary Therapies in Nursing and Midwifery 8(4):204–210

Long L, Huntley A, Ernst E 2001 Which complementary and alternative therapies benefit which conditions? A survey of the opinions of 223 professional organizations. Complementary Therapies in Medicine 9(3):178–185

Potter R 2002 Evidence points to effectiveness of Bowen for frozen shoulder. Physiotherapy Frontline 8(7):16

### Resources

Bowen Association UK: www.bowen-technique.co.uk

## Chiropractic

*Description*

Chiropractic, an offshoot of osteopathy, is a manipulative therapy developed during the 19th century by Daniel Palmer (1845–1913), the term originating from the Greek *cheir* (hands) and *praktikos* (practice). Palmer believed that most medical problems result from misalignments of the musculoskeletal system, notably the vertebrae or from subluxation, altered alignment, impaired movement integrity and/or physiological dysfunction, which leads to nerve entrapment and disruption of nerve transmissions.

Specific techniques used in chiropractic include: high velocity–low amplitude (HVLA) thrusts over segments or groups of segments of the body; leverage in which a thrust is performed with counter-stabilization to prevent loss of force; impulse-movement using a short quick thrust; and recoil, in which the force of the practitioner's arms, chest and hands facilitates the thrust, followed by recoil of the hands from the patient's vertebrae. Techniques for specific conditions include: the Cox/flexion-distraction, a traction/mobilization technique, particularly useful for intervertebral disc pathology; the Pierce–Stillwagon technique for pelvic and cervical spine dysfunctions; the Thompson technique to correct pelvic dysfunction, particularly if there is a discrepancy in leg length; the Logan basic, in which sacral dysfunctions are treated by using fascial release techniques; and the Webster technique for converting a breech-presenting fetus to cephalic. Another technique, chiroenergetics, aids release of muscular tension associated with suppressed psychological traumas.

There are various types of chiropractic. The Gonstead technique uses high velocity–low amplitude thrusts directly on the locus of impeded movement. McTimoney chiropractic, a particularly gentle form suitable for babies and the elderly, developed by John McTimoney in the 1950s, uses a technique called the toggle-recoil to change the tension surrounding a joint with a rapid thrust followed by immediate release. In the Meric method it is believed that the third thoracic vertebra is the primary centre of subluxation, for which high velocity–low amplitude thrusts are applied.

Evidence:    Chiropractic is most commonly used for musculoskeletal problems notably back and neck pain and there is a fair amount of clinical evidence, at least in the form of case studies and single case cohorts. The therapy has also been found to be effective for the treatment of soft tissue conditions triggered or exacerbated by musculoskeletal misalignment, e.g. duodenal ulcer.

Safety: Chiropractors are statutorily regulated by the General Chiropractic Council and, as such, must adhere to a code of practice which requires them to remain up-to-date in their knowledge and skills, therefore practitioners should be aware of relevant contraindications and precautions to treatment. Chiropractic is not suitable for people with osteoporosis, advanced degenerative joint disease or bone metastases. Initial adverse reactions include temporary dizziness, local discomfort or numbness or radiating pain. Some reports of very rare complications include stroke and neurological damage.

## Bibliography

Beattie P F, Nelson R M, Michener L A et al 2008 Outcomes after a prone lumbar traction protocol for patients with activity-limiting low back pain: a prospective case series study. Archives of Physical Medicine and Rehabilitation 89(2):269–274

Cassidy J D, Boyle E, Côté P et al 2008 Risk of vertebrobasilar stroke and chiropractic care: results of a population-based case-control and case-crossover study. Spine 33(Suppl):S176 S183

Jonas W, Levin S 1999 Essentials of Complementary Alternative Medicine. Lippincott, Baltimore

Kurbanyan K, Lessell S 2008 Intracranial hypotension and abducens palsy following upper spinal manipulation. British Journal of Ophthalmology 92(1):153–155

Livdans-Forret A B, Harvey P J, Larkin-Thier S M 2007 Menorrhagia: a synopsis of management focusing on herbal and nutritional supplements and chiropractic. Journal of the Canadian Chiropractic Association 51(4):235–246

Maiers M J, Hartvigsen J, Schulz C et al 2007 Chiropractic and exercise for seniors with low back pain or neck pain: the design of two randomized clinical trials. BMC Musculoskeletal Disorders 8:94

McHardy A, Hoskins W, Pollard H et al 2008 Chiropractic treatment of upper extremity conditions: a systematic review. Journal of Manipulative and Physiological Therapeutics 31(2):146–159

Myers S S, Phillips R S, Davis R B et al 2008 Patient expectations as predictors of outcome in patients with acute low back pain. Journal of General Internal Medicine 23(2):148–153

Pistolese R A 2002 The Webster technique: a chiropractic technique with obstetric implications. Journal of Manipulative and Physiological Therapeutics 25(6):E1–E9

Rasmussen H R, Terndrup P G, Myburgh C et al 2008 Pain perception in patients with intermittent low back pain. Journal of Manipulative and Physiological Therapeutics 31(2):127–129

Rubinstein S M, Leboeuf-Yde C, Knol D L et al 2008 Predictors of adverse events following chiropractic care for patients with neck pain. Journal of Manipulative and Physiological Therapeutics 31(2):94–103

Ruiz-Sáez M, Fernández-de-las-Peñas C, Blanco C R et al 2007 Changes in pressure pain sensitivity in latent myofascial trigger points in the upper trapezius muscle after a cervical spine manipulation in pain-free subjects. Journal of Manipulative and Physiological Therapeutics 30(8):578–583

Theberge N 2008 The integration of chiropractors into healthcare teams: a case study from sport medicine. Sociology of Health and Illness 30(1):19–34

### Resources

British Chiropractic Council: www.chiropractic-uk.co.uk
Chiropractic Patients Association: www.chiropatients.org.uk
General Chiropractic Council: www.gcc-uk.org
McTimoney Chiropractic Association: www.mctimoney-chiropractic.org

## Feldenkrais

*Description*

Feldenkrais was developed by Moshe Feldenkrais and offers a process of body re-education which aims to make clients aware of the body in motion, to improve flexibility and to enhance well-being through touch and gentle manipulation. This is achieved either on a one-to-one basis (during which individually tailored touch and manipulation are referred to as 'functional integration') or in group sessions (in which exercises are performed to develop body awareness and flexibility, i.e. 'awareness through movement').

Evidence:    There is some suggestion for the use of this technique for chronic pain. It may also have a place in the treatment of people with cerebral palsy, possibly facilitating improved movement.

Safety:    No information regarding safety, contraindications or precautions was found.

### Bibliography

Buchanan P A, Ulrich B D 2001 The Feldenkrais Method: a dynamic approach to changing motor behavior. Research Questions Exercise Sport 72(4):315–323

Gard G 2005 Body awareness therapy for patients with fibromyalgia and chronic pain. Disability Rehabilitation 27(12):725–728

Ives J C 2003 Comments on 'the Feldenkrais Method: a dynamic approach to changing motor behavior'. Research Quarterly for Exercise and Sport 74(2): 116–123, discussion 124–126

Jain S, Janssen K, DeCelle S 2004 Alexander technique and Feldenkrais method: a critical overview. Physical Medicine and Rehabilitation Clinics of North America 15(4):811–825

Liptak G S 2005 Complementary and alternative therapies for cerebral palsy. Mental Retardation and Developmental Disabilities Research Reviews 11(2):156–163

Maher C G 2004 Effective physical treatment for chronic low back pain. Orthopedic Clinics of North America 35(1):57–64

Mehling W E, DiBlasi Z, Hecht F 2005 Bias control in trials of bodywork: a review of methodological issues. Journal of Alternative and Complementary Medicine 11(2):333–342

Schlinger M 2006 Feldenkrais Method, Alexander Technique and yoga – body awareness therapy in the performing arts. Physical Medical Rehabilitation Clinics North America 17(4):865–875

### Resources

Feldenkrais Guild UK: www.feldenkrais.co.uk

## Heller work

### Description

Heller work was developed by Joseph Heller in the 1970s and is based on the concepts of deep tissue massage which unblocks the body; verbal dialogue to assess emotional holding patterns; and movement re-education to correct postural misalignment. It is believed that memory is seated not only in the brain but also in the muscles and tissues of the body, so that adjusting the body at the physical level can also produce an emotional effect, while conversely, addressing emotional issues assists in the amelioration of physical conditions. The therapy follows a rigid structure of 11 sessions with follow-up advice and exercises.

Evidence: No studies relating to the efficacy or safety of Heller work could be found.

Safety: No information regarding safety, contraindications or precautions was found.

Bibliography

Moran D S, Pandolf K B, Heled Y et al; US Army Research Institute of Environmental Medicine; Natick, Massachusetts 01760-5007, USA 2003 Combined environmental stress and physiological strain indices for physical training guidelines. Journal of Basic and Clinical Physiology and Pharmacology 14(1): 17–30

Resources

Heller work: www.hellerwork-europe.com

## Massage

### Description

The concept of massage has evolved into a number of interventions and techniques, ranging from gentle soothing movements to deep massage techniques. The most commonly used, movements include: effleurage, a deep or superficial stroking using the palmar surface of the hand to aid relaxation and circulation; pétrissage, a circular kneading movement with fingers and thumbs to stimulate muscles, improve lymphatic drainage and circulation and to break up adhesions; stimulating movements such as friction and percussion (brisk hacking or tapping with the fingertips); tapotement, in which rapid, repeated taps with the palms, sides or cupped hands are used to stimulate and revive; and vibration, the use of small superficial rapid movements of the fingertips or palms. Massage is incorporated into many traditional systems of medicine, including Japanese anma, Chinese tuina, Swedish massage, Indian head massage, Thai yoga massage and Hawaiian lomi lomi. It is also the foundation for many other bodywork therapies, as detailed in this section.

Evidence:   Massage has been shown to aid relaxation, ease pain and discomfort and improve well-being. Several studies with preterm babies demonstrate its effectiveness in improving weight gain, intellectual ability and overall prognosis; it is also of value in treating children with attention deficit hyperactivity disorder (ADHD) and depressed adolescents. In pregnancy, massage enhances fetal well-being and improves labour outcomes. In adults, it is beneficial in reducing blood pressure, stimulating excretory processes and for general relaxation.

Safety: The deep relaxation induced by massage means that it should only be used with extreme caution in epileptics, especially those in whom a fit may be triggered by sedation as opposed to stimulation. This factor also suggests that massage, particularly that which specifically induces relaxation, may be contraindicated for people with psychosis or hallucinations, although it may be of benefit during a non-active period of illness. Direct massage over areas of thrombosis, varicosities, fracture or tumour should be avoided but generalized massage is acceptable for people with these conditions, with caution. As massage has a warming effect, it should not be performed during a febrile episode. During the first trimester of pregnancy, brisk massage of the heels is probably best avoided, as this area corresponds to the reflexology zone for the pelvis; abdominal massage should be avoided if the placenta is situated on the anterior wall of the uterus or if there is any history of antepartum bleeding; and breast massage may be uncomfortable or rejected due to leakage of colostrum.

## Bibliography

Beider S, Mahrer N E, Gold J I 2007 Pediatric massage therapy: an overview for clinicians. Pediatric Clinics of North America 54(6):1025–1041

Cambron J A, Dexheimer J, Coe P et al 2007 Side-effects of massage therapy: a cross-sectional study of 100 clients. Journal of Alternative and Complementary Medicine 13(8):793–796

Coelho H F, Boddy K, Ernst E 2008 Massage therapy for the treatment of depression: a systematic review. International Journal of Clinical Practice 62(2):325–333

Ejindu A 2007 The effects of foot and facial massage on sleep induction, blood pressure, pulse and respiratory rate: crossover pilot study. Complementary Therapies in Clinical Practice 13(4):266–275

Frey Law L A, Evans S, Knudtson J et al 2008 Massage reduces pain perception and hyperalgesia in experimental muscle pain: a randomized, controlled trial. Journal of Pain 9(8):714–721

Hughes D, Ladas E, Rooney D et al 2008 Massage therapy as a supportive care intervention for children with cancer. Oncology Nursing Forum 35(3):431–442

Imamura M, Furlan A D, Dryden T et al 2008 Evidence-informed management of chronic low back pain with massage. Spine Journal 8(1):121–133

Jabr F 2007 Massive pulmonary embolism after leg massage. American Journal of Physical Medicine and Rehabilitation 86(8):691

Kaye A D, Kaye A J, Swinford J et al 2008 The effect of deep-tissue massage therapy on blood pressure and heart rate. Journal of Alternative and Complementary Medicine 14(2):125–128

Mitchinson A R, Kim H M, Rosenberg J M et al 2007 Acute postoperative pain management using massage as an adjuvant therapy: a randomized trial. Archives of Surgery 142(12):1158–1167

O'Higgins M, St James Roberts I, Glover V 2007 Postnatal depression and mother and infant outcomes after infant massage. Journal of Affective Disorders 109 (1–2):189–192

Robershawe P 2007 Massage improves sleep in infants with low birth weight. Journal of Australian Traditional Medicine Society 13(1):33

Robershawe P 2007 Regular massage in late pregnancy decreases pain in labour. Journal of Australian Traditional Medicine Society 13(1):7

Russell N C, Sumler S S, Beinhorn C M et al 2008 Role of massage therapy in cancer care. Journal of Alternative and Complementary Medicine 14(2): 209–214

Stringer J, Swindell R, Dennis M 2008 Massage in patients undergoing intensive chemotherapy reduces serum cortisol and prolactin. Psychooncology 26 Feb

---

Resources

---

General Council for Massage Therapy: www.gcmt-uk.org

## Metamorphic technique

*Description*

Metamorphic technique has its origins in reflexology and was developed by Robert St John (1912–1996), a British naturopath and reflexologist. The technique involves a light touch to the reflex points in the foot, hands and head which relate to the spinal column in order to bring about transformations in the energy patterns. Metamorphic technique was originally called 'prenatal therapy' the aim of which was to remove energy blockages, thought to have occurred while the person was still *in utero*, by activating reflexology points relating to the spinal column which are also said to correspond to the various stages of fetal life. These energy blocks are thought to have manifested themselves as patterns of behaviour and the aim of therapy was to release them. Subsequently, another therapist, Gaston Saint-Pierre, suggested that treatment should aim to dissolve rather than unblock the energy blockages.

Evidence: No contemporary clinical research on safety or efficacy could be found; some early accounts reported the apparent success of Metamorphic technique in aiding socialization and improving physical interactions of children with autism, but these have not been included here since no more recent reports have been found.

Safety: No information regarding safety, contraindications or precautions was found.

### Bibliography

No recent professional literature was found.

### Resources

Metamorphic Association: www.metamorphicassociation.org

## Neuromuscular therapy

*Description*

This therapy involves treatment of somatic dysfunctions (areas of tenderness and limited movement) with a combination of effleurage, pétrissage for specific muscles or friction with strain and counter strain techniques.

Evidence: No clinical evidence was found on the therapy as a whole, although there is some evidence on its individual components, i.e. massage and strain/counter strain techniques.

Safety: No information regarding safety, contraindications or precautions was found.

### Bibliography

No professional literature was found.

## Osteopathy

*Description*

Osteopathy is a manipulative therapy founded by Dr Andrew Taylor Still, based on the principle that the foundation of good health lies in correct alignment of the musculoskeletal system. Misalignment of the musculoskeletal system, due to injury, trauma, disease or genetic factors, places stress and tension on the body, leading to further disease and disorder in related organs or systems. Techniques used include gentle passive movements, such as strain and counterstrain to treat muscle spasm, myofascial soft tissue release and lymphatic drainage, in which movements similar to effleurage are directed towards the heart to increase lymphatic return. Other techniques include high velocity–low amplitude movements, using short quick thrusts (high velocity) over short distances (low amplitude) against resistance; and muscle energy technique, involving the tensing and releasing of certain muscles to induce relaxation.

An off-shoot of osteopathy is cranial osteopathy, developed by William Sutherland and based on his assertion that the cerebrospinal fluid pulses rhythmically at 12–15 beats/min: disturbance of this pulsation can lead to imbalances within the body. Treatment involves tiny manipulations of the skull, spinal column and sacrum and manipulation of the soft tissues, fluid and membrane of the craniosacral system. Cranial osteopaths are always qualified osteopaths, whereas those who practise a similar technique called cranio-sacral therapy, a further development of Sutherland's work brought to the UK by the American osteopath Dr J. Upledger, may be either osteopaths or physiotherapists or lay practitioners.

Evidence:    Several trials demonstrate the effectiveness of osteopathy primarily in the treatment of musculoskeletal disorders, disability and chronic pain, specifically back pain. There is some evidence that craniosacral therapy can be useful for treating colic in babies and that it may have a role in the treatment of dementia in the elderly. However, systematic reviews have shown variable results, with osteopathy being viewed positively, but highlighting that there is insufficient evidence to support the use of craniosacral therapy.

Safety:    Osteopaths are statutorily regulated by the General Osteopathic Council and, as such, must adhere to a code of practice which requires them to remain up-to-date in their knowledge and skills, therefore, practitioners should be aware of relevant contraindications and precautions to treatment. Osteopathy is not suitable for people with osteoporosis, advanced degenerative joint disease or bone metastases. Initial adverse reactions include temporary dizziness, local discomfort or numbness or radiating pain. Some reports of very rare complications include stroke and neurological damage.

## Bibliography

De-Angelo N, Gordin V 2004 Treatment of patients with arthritis related pain. Journal of the American Osteopathic Association 104(11 Suppl 8):s2–s5

Downey P A, Barbano T, Kapur-Wadhwa R et al 2006 Craniosacral therapy: the effects of cranial manipulation on intracranial pressure and cranial bone movement. Journal of Orthopaedic and Sports Physical Therapy 36(11): 845–853

Duncan B, Barton L, Edmonds D et al 2006 The somatic connection. Osteopathic manipulative treatment and acupuncture proved therapeutic benefit to children with spastic cerebral palsy. Journal of the American Osteopathic Association 106(7):381

Eisenhart A, Gaeta T, Yens D 2003 Osteopathic manipulative treatment in the emergency department for patients with acute ankle injuries. Journal of the American Osteopathic Association 103(9):417–421

Gerdner L A, Hart L K, Zimmerman M B 2008 Craniosacral still point technique: exploring its effects in individuals with dementia. Journal of Gerontological Nursing 34(3):36–45

Gillespie B R 2008 Case study in pediatric asthma: the corrective aspect of craniosacral fascial therapy. Explore (NY) 4(1):48–51

Green C, Martin C W, Bassett K et al 1999 A systematic review of craniosacral therapy: biological plausibility, assessment reliability and clinical effectiveness. Complementary Therapies in Medicine 7(4):201–207

Harvey E, Burton A, Moffett J et al 2003 Spinal manipulation for low-back pain: a treatment package agreed to by the UK chiropractic, osteopathy and physiotherapy professional associations. Manual Therapies 8(1):46–51

Licciardone J 2004 The unique role of osteopathic physicians in treating patients with low back pain. Journal of the American Osteopathic Association 104(Suppl): s13–s18

Licciardone J 2007 Responding to the challenge of clinically relevant osteopathic research: efficacy and beyond. International Journal of Osteopathic Medicine 10(1):3–7

Licciardone J, Stoll S, Fulda K et al 2003 Osteopathic manipulative treatment for chronic low back pain: a randomised controlled trial. Spine 28(13):1355–1362

McManus V, Gliksten M 2007 The use of craniosacral therapy in a physically impaired population in a disability service in southern Ireland. Journal of Alternative and Complementary Medicine 13(9):929–930

Nourbakhsh M R, Fearon F J 2008 The effect of oscillating-energy manual therapy on lateral epicondylitis: a randomized, placebo-control, double-blinded study. Journal of Hand Therapy 21(1):4–13

Potter L, McCarthy C, Oldham J 2005 Physiological effects of spinal manipulation: a review of proposed theories. Physical Therapy Review 10(3):163–170

Tsao J C, Meldrum M, Kim S C et al 2007 Treatment preferences for CAM in children with chronic pain. Evidence-Based Complementary and Alternative Medicine 4(3):367–374

Weng-Lim K 2006 Infantile colic: a critical appraisal of the literature from an osteopathic perspective. International Journal of Osteopathy 9(3):94–102

### Resources

General Osteopathic Council: www.goc.org www.osteopathy.org.uk
Chartered Society of Physiotherapists: www.csp.org.uk
National Back Pain Association: www.backpain.org

## Reflexology

*Description*

Reflexology is a generic term referring to the use of one small part of the body which is said to represent a map of the whole. It is thought to have been used by the Chinese over 5000 years ago and has been recorded in Assyria, India and Egypt. Generally, reflexology is delivered via the feet, but the hands, face, ear, back and tongue can also be used. Although the treatment is relaxing – and can be used for relaxation, relief of stress, tension and anxiety – it is not simply a massage, but utilizes precise pressure points which are thought to reflect back to the organs they represent, possibly via neural pathways, although contemporary theories focus more on the meridian approach similar to Oriental medicine. There are various maps and charts in use; contemporary academics aim to explore the variations between these different charts. Reflexology can be used to restore and maintain homeostasis and is commonly given as a general relaxing session, but in clinical reflexology, specific conditions can also be treated.

There are various styles of reflexology. Reflex zone therapy, developed by Hanne Marquardt from the zone therapy work by William Fitzgerald, an American ear, nose and throat surgeon, works on the principle of both longitudinal and horizontal zones on the feet, corresponding to different sections of the body; treatment intends to focus on the causes of disease, rather than just the symptoms. Reflex zone therapy takes a more reductionist, clinical approach to treatment than generalized reflexology, some forms of which have a more esoteric approach based on the principles of energy medicine. Chi reflexology and Five Element reflexology focus more specifically on the meridians of Chinese medicine; upright reflexology utilizes the dorsal surfaces of the feet with the client in the upright position; Vacuflex™ reflexology involves the use of a special inflatable 'boot' via which pressure can be applied to the reflex zones in the feet.

Evidence: Reflexology has been shown to ease pain, perhaps via the gate control theory, although some have questioned this, believing it to be a placebo effect. Other studies have favourably compared reflexology to standard pharmacological treatments for conditions such as headache, labour pain and backache. Symptoms of multiple sclerosis, irritable bowel syndrome, constipation and premenstrual syndrome have also responded well to reflexology. The claim by reflexologists that they can identify changing physiology and potential pathology has not been confirmed in formal studies, which suggests that practitioners tend to 'over-diagnose' identifying conditions which do not actually exist.

Safety: There are several contraindications and precautions to reflexology treatment. Care should be taken when treating diabetics, as over-stimulation of the foot zone relating to the pancreas may theoretically trigger a hypoglycaemic attack. Treatment is completely contraindicated in epileptics, as the deep relaxation from treatment could trigger a fit. Those with deep vein thrombosis should not receive foot reflexology, although hand or ear treatment is possible; caution should be used when treating clients with varicose veins. Reflexology should also be used with caution in individuals who have foreign bodies in situ, as there is a theoretical possibility that these could be moved out of position, for example, a pacemaker, intrauterine contraceptive device or even abnormal pathology such as renal calculi or gallstones. Treatment is warming and should therefore not be used on patients with hyper-pyrexia. During pregnancy, treatment should generally only be given by practitioners who are either midwives or who have undertaken specialist preparation to treat pregnant clients. It is safe for children. Cancer patients should be treated with caution and may only be able to tolerate sessions of short duration.

## Bibliography

Bishop E, McKinnon E, Weir E et al 2003 Reflexology in the management of encopresis and chronic constipation. Paediatric Nursing 15(3):20–21

Brendstrup E, Launso L, Eriksen L 1997 Headaches and Reflexological Treatment, 4th edn. Association of Reflexologists' Research Reports, London

Brown C A, Lido C 2008 Reflexology treatment for patients with lower limb amputations and phantom limb pain. An exploratory pilot study. Complementary Therapies in Clinical Practice 14(2):124–131

Deborah M 2007 Reflexology and integrative imagery: promoting healing in patients, families and practitioners. Beginnings 27(4):6–7

Hodgson N, Andersen S 2008 The clinical efficacy of reflexology in nursing home residents with dementia. Journal of Alternative and Complementary Medicine 14(3):269–275

Kim Y S, Kim M Z, Jeong I S 2004 The effect of self-foot reflexology on the relief of premenstrual syndrome and dysmenorrhea in high school girls. Taehan Kanho Hakhoe Chi 34(5):801–808

Mackereth P, Tiran D (eds) 2002 Clinical Reflexology: A Guide for Health Professionals. Elsevier, London

Mollart L 2003 Single-blind trial addressing the differential effects of two reflexology techniques versus rest, on ankle and foot oedema in late pregnancy. Complementary Therapies in Nursing and Midwifery 9(4):203–208

Mur E, Schmidseder J, Egger I et al 2001 Influence of reflex zone therapy of the feet on intestinal blood flow measured by color Doppler sonography. Forschende Komplementärmedizin und Klassische Naturheilkunde 8(2):86–89

Quinn F, Hughes C M, Baxter G D 2008 Reflexology in the management of low back pain: a pilot randomised controlled trial. Complementary Therapies in Medicine 16(1):3–8

Tiran D, Chummun H 2005 The physiological basis of reflexology and its use as a diagnostic tool. Complementary Therapies in Clinical Practice 11(1):58–64

Tovey P 2002 A single-blind trial of reflexology for irritable bowel syndrome. British Journal of General Practice 52(474):19–23

White A R, Williamson J, Hart A et al 2000 A blinded investigation into the accuracy of reflexology charts. Complementary Therapies in Medicine 8(3):166–172

Williamson J, White A, Hart A et al 2002 Randomised controlled trial of reflexology for menopausal symptoms. British Journal of Obstetrics and Gynaecology 109(9):1050–1055

Resources

Association of Reflexologists: www.aor.org.uk
Reflexology Forum: www.reflexologyforum.org

## Rolfing

*Description*

Rolfing (also called structural re-integration therapy) involves the use of deep massage techniques to loosen and relax the fascia and muscles, together with re-education of the client to help him/her correct body misalignment and maladaptive movement patterns. It was developed by Ida Rolf (1896–1979), a biochemist who studied a range of complementary therapies when treatment of her own medical condition fell short of her expectations. A key concept is the relationship between the client and the gravitational force acting upon them – a state of equilibrium should be attained so that potential energy (form) is in direct proportion to kinetic energy (function), the balance being equivalent to the amount of available energy in the body. If the person has poor posture, more energy is needed to perform the necessary functions. The system is influenced by three key principles: the osteopathic belief that structure determines function; the homeopathic emphasis on the integration of a person's mental, emotional and physical factors; and the yogic focus on lengthening and strengthening positions to achieve a balanced body. Treatment involves 10 sessions during which the connective tissue system is lengthened using a series of myofascial release techniques. As treatment progresses, emotional components may be manifest and the unblocking of emotional processes is seen as an integral part of the treatment.

Evidence:   No clinical evidence was found.

Safety:   No information regarding safety, contraindications or precautions was found.

Bibliography

Mehling W E, DiBlasi Z, Hecht F 2005 Bias control in trials of bodywork: a review
of methodological issues. Journal of Alternative and Complementary Medicine
11(2):333–342

Resources

Rolf Institute: www.rolf.org

## Tragerwork

*Description*

Tragerwork is a system of body re-education to enable clients to un-learn dysfunctional mental and physical habits, using gentle, rhythmic, pushing, pulling, rocking and stretching of the body to loosen muscles and joints and increase the range of movements, together with enhanced relaxation – psychophysical integration – which includes dance-like exercises called mentastics to increase body awareness.

Evidence:    No clinical evidence was found.

Safety:    No information regarding safety, contraindications or precautions was found.

Bibliography

Mehling W E, DiBlasi Z, Hecht F 2005 Bias control in trials of bodywork: a review
of methodological issues. Journal of Alternative and Complementary Medicine
11(2):333–342

Resources

Trager International: www.trager.com

## Trigger point therapy

*Description*

Trigger point therapy (also called deep tissue therapy, myotherapy or manual ischaemic compression therapy) is a manual therapy based on the principle that, following injury, damaged tissue leads to the development of trigger points, areas of localized hypersensitivity which are tender when compressed. This gives rise to stiffness, restricted movement, fatigue and referred pain. The trigger points can be activated if the muscle is over-used or there is excess emotional or physical stress, resulting in spasm, deep muscular ache or sharp disabling pain leading to a spasm/pain/spasm cycle. Treatment involves deactivation of the trigger point and myomassage to relieve the spasm.

Evidence:   Recent evidence supports the use of this technique for headache and myofascial pain.

Safety:   No information was available regarding safety. No evidence of any contraindications was found.

Bibliography

Cummings M, Baldry P 2007 Regional myofascial pain: diagnosis and management. Best Practice Research Clinical Rheumatology 21(2):367–387

Fernández-de-las-Peñas C, Cleland J A, Cuadrado M L et al 2008 Predictor variables for identifying patients with chronic tension-type headache who are likely to achieve short-term success with muscle trigger point therapy. Cephalalgia 28(3):264–275

Ga H, Koh H J, Choi J H et al 2007 Intramuscular and nerve root stimulation vs lidocaine injection to trigger points in myofascial pain syndrome. Journal of Rehabilitation Medicine 39(5):374–378

Itoh K, Hirota S, Katsumi Y et al 2008 Trigger point acupuncture for treatment of knee osteoarthritis – a preliminary RCT for a pragmatic trial. Acupuncture in Medicine 26(1):17–26

Lavelle E D, Lavelle W, Smith H S 2007 Myofascial trigger points. Anesthesiology Clinics 25(4):841–851, vii–iii

Malanga G, Wolff E 2008 Evidence-informed management of chronic low back pain with trigger point injections. Spine Journal 8(1):243–252

## Breathwork therapies

*Description*

Breathwork is a collective term for several therapies which aim to heal through the medium of breathing exercises and techniques, with breath control, to maximize the body's physical potential and to clear and clarify the mind.

## Buteyko

*Description*

This therapy was devised by Dr Konstantin Buteyko in Moscow and aims primarily to alleviate asthma symptoms, but has also been used for allergies, hyperventilation, emphysema and chronic obstructive pulmonary disease. The system aims to teach the person to breathe very shallowly, avoiding deep inspirations, both at the onset of and during an asthma attack thus raising alveolar carbon dioxide levels.

Evidence:   Results from some clinical trials indicate a reduction in inhaler use in asthmatics but the technique is generally not supported by the Cochrane Review team.

Safety:   No information was found regarding safety, contraindications or precautions. However, conventional healthcare professionals should advise patients that this therapy should not be used as a substitute for orthodox medical treatment in life-threatening situations.

Bibliography

Al-Delaimy W, Hay S, Gain K et al 2001 The effects of carbon dioxide on exercise induced asthma: an unlikely explanation for the effects of Buteyko breathing training. Medical Journal of Australia 174(2):72–77

Bowler S, Green A, Mitchell C 1998 Buteyko breathing techniques in asthma: a blinded randomised trial. Medical Journal of Australia 169(11–12):575–578

Bruton A, Lewith G 2005 The Buteyko breathing technique for asthma: a review. Complementary Therapies in Medicine 13(1):41–46

Courtney R, Cohen M 2008 Investigating the claims of Konstantin Buteyko, MD, PhD: the relationship of breath holding time to end tidal $CO_2$ and other proposed measures of dysfunctional breathing. Journal of Alternative and Complementary Medicine 14(2):115–123

Cowie R L, Conley D P, Underwood M F et al 2008 A randomised controlled trial of the Buteyko technique as an adjunct to conventional management of asthma. Respiratory Medicine 102(5):726–732

Holloway E, Ram F 2000 Breathing exercises for asthma. Cochrane Database of Systematic Reviews(3), CD001277

Kuiper D 2001 Dysfunctional breathing and asthma. Trial shows benefits of Buteyko breathing techniques. British Medical Journal 323(7313):631–632

McHugh P, Duncan B, Houghton F 2006 Buteyko breathing technique and asthma in children: a case series. New Zealand Medical Journal 119(1234):U1988

McHugh P, Aitcheson F, Duncan B et al 2004 Buteyko: an effective complementary therapy. New Zealand Medical Journal 117(1189):U781

Opat A J, Cohen M M, Bailey M J et al 2000 A clinical trial of the Buteyko breathing technique in asthma as taught by a video. Journal of Asthma 37(7):557–564

Shaw A, Thompson E A, Sharp D 2006 Complementary therapy use by patients and parents of children with asthma and the implications for NHS care: a qualitative study. BMC Health Services Research 6:76

Thomas S 2004 Buteyko: a useful tool in the management of asthma? International Journal of Therapeutic Rehabilitation 11(10):476–480

White A 2001 The Buteyko explanation of asthma does not gain strong support. Focus on Alternative and Complementary Therapies 6(2):132–133

### Resources

Buteyko: www.buteyko.co.uk

## Holotropic breathwork

*Description*

This therapy combines breathing exercises, art and music to alter consciousness and encourage spiritual development.

Evidence: There is some suggestion that it may be useful for common psychiatric disorders including anxiety and depression.

Safety: No information regarding safety or any contraindications was found.

### Bibliography

Rhinewine J P, Williams O J 2007 Holotropic breathwork: the potential role of a prolonged, voluntary hyperventilation procedure as an adjunct to psychotherapy. Journal of Alternative and Complementary Medicine 13(7):771–776

## Rebirthing

*Description*

This modality was instigated by Leonard Orr in the 1960s when he noticed that hot water and relaxation induced a sense of being 'somewhere else'. He developed a system to harness this feeling, using connected breathing, which apparently leads to a complete rebirthing experience, enabling people to address childhood issues of self esteem or lack of assertiveness. Later he decided that hot baths were not necessary for the process and that the key to success was in the breathing technique. Contemporary rebirthing requires 10 sessions with a rebirther and thereafter, people can rebirth themselves.

Evidence:    No evidence from clinical trials was found, but surveys of attitudes to complementary medicine and its use among the general public occasionally mention rebirthing as a popular therapy.

Safety:    No information regarding safety, efficacy, contraindications and precautions was found.

### Bibliography

Begg D 2001 A guide to rebirthing. Connections 39:30–32

Malassiotis A, Margulies A, Fernandez-Ortega P et al 2005 Complementary and alternative medicine use in patients with haematological malignancies in Europe. Complementary Therapies in Clinical Practice 11(2):105–110

### Resources

British Rebirth Society: www.rebirthingbreathwork.co.uk

## Vivation

*Description*

Vivation claims to teach the client how to be happy – happiness being regarded as a skill which can be learned – and involves the integration of negative experiences in order that they may become positive, through circular breathing to re-energize the energy patterns. Complete relaxation as an aid to reducing resistance; awareness in detail through interpretation of the feelings experienced; and integration into ecstasy – changing the context of the feeling and transforming it to a positive experience. This aims to focus on the person's willingness to experience the integration.

Evidence:    None found.

Safety:    No information regarding efficacy, safety, contraindications or precautions was found.

### Bibliography

No professional literature was found.

### Resources

Vivation: www.vivation-uk.com

# C

## Cancer therapies

*Description*

Numerous therapies claiming to treat or even to cure cancer have been developed over the years by individuals and organizations, many before the advent of modern chemotherapy. These therapies and interventions are still in demand, largely in response to people's disenchantment with orthodox medicine, although few have been shown to be effective or safe in clinical trials. It is, however, important for conventional healthcare professionals to appreciate that cancer patients may resort to alternatives, usually as an adjunct, but unfortunately, sometimes as a replacement for orthodox medical treatment and occasionally, as a desperate last resort when conventional medicine can do no more.

Evidence: Many of the therapies and self-help strategies which claim to treat cancer or to assist in the alleviation of pathological or treatment-induced symptoms, are scientifically unproven, although some have become so popular that there appears to be a considerable placebo effect, which can be beneficial in its own right. Many cancer patients also use a variety of accepted and evidence-based complementary therapies for relaxation, including massage, aromatherapy, reflexology and others and these have been considered elsewhere in this book. This section deals with some of the more obscure therapies and therefore much of the information has been collated from various consumer websites and voluntary support organizations.

Safety: While there are specific safety concerns related to some of the alternative cancer treatments, the over-riding general concern is that patients risk delay in obtaining proven orthodox medical treatments, for which, while they can be extremely unpleasant, there may be a chance of a reasonable prognosis. Alternatively, concurrent use of some of the alternatives with orthodox medical treatment may either produce interactions, for example between herbal remedies and prescribed pharmacological preparations or produce apparent side-effects, in the form of a healing crisis response to therapies such as homeopathic remedies, which may complicate the overall clinical picture. Nurses should ask cancer patients about their use of any alternatives, including specialist diets and consider how their choices may impact on their overall well-being. It should be remembered that, in the UK, it is against the law to claim to 'cure' cancer – and those labelled as such, at the very least, risk giving patients unrealistic expectations of their chances of full recovery.

### Bibliography

Cassileth B 1999 Complementary and alternative cancer medicine. Journal of Clinical Oncology 17(Suppl):44–52

Davis P 2006 Conversations with a nurse in cancer complementary and alternative medicine. Clinical Journal of Oncology Nursing 10(6):829–830

Ernst E, Boddy K 2006 CAM cancer diets. Focus on Alternative and Complementary Therapies 11(2):91–95

Lee C 2004 Clinical trials in cancer, Part II Biomedical, complementary and alternative medicine: significant issues. Clinical Journal of Oncology Nursing 8(6):670–674

Maritess C, Small S, Waltz-Hill M 2005 Alternative nutrition therapies in cancer patients. Seminars in Oncology Nursing 21(3):173–176

Schmidt K 2002 CAM and the desperate call for cancer cures and alleviation. What can websites offer cancer patients? Complementary Therapies in Medicine 10(3):170–180

Vickers A 2001 Unconventional therapies for cancer and cancer related symptoms. Lancet Oncology 2(4):226–232

Vickers A, Kuo J, Cassileth-Barrie R 2006 Unconventional anti cancer agents: systematic review of clinical trials. Journal of Clinical Oncology 24(1):136–140

Weitzman S 2008 Complementary and alternative (CAM) dietary therapies for cancer. Pediatric Blood and Cancer 50(Suppl):494–497

## Penny Brohn Cancer Centre nutritional approach

*Description*

The Penny Brohn Cancer Centre (formerly the Bristol Cancer Help Centre) offers an approach to nutrition for cancer patients which was originally vegan, emphasizing whole foods, fruits and vegetables (up to 10 portions daily), raw cereals and essential fatty acids. More recently, the approach has been modified and now includes eggs, organic fish and poultry, while avoiding alcohol, caffeine, salt, dairy produce, sugar and red meat.

Evidence:   No recent clinical evidence was found.

Safety:   The original diet lacked essential nutrients but the contemporary modified version is rather more balanced. While this diet may be of benefit to complement other conventional treatments, it should not be taken as a 'cure' approach.

### Bibliography

No recent professional literature was found.

### Resources

Penny Brohn Cancer Centre: www.pennybrohncancercare.org

## Budwig's oil protein diet

*Description*

This diet was devised by Dr Johanna Budwig, a German biochemist, physician and expert on fats and oils and comprises fruit, fruit juices and a mixture of flaxseed oil and curd cheese.

Evidence:   No professional literature was found.

Safety:   No information was available regarding safety, contraindications and precautions. The nutritional status of patients relying on this diet during their cancer journey may become imbalanced.

### Bibliography

No professional literature was found.

## Cantron

*Description*

Cantron (formerly Cancell) is a product claimed to cure cancer by 'lowering the voltage of cells by 20%' causing autolysis of cancer cells which can then be replaced by normal cells. It consists of inositol, nitric acid, sodium sulphite, potassium hydroxide, sulphuric acid and catechol. Manufacturers claim it changes its energy depending on atmospheric vibrations.

Evidence:   None found.

Safety:   No information regarding safety or contraindications was found. There is no evidence that this remedy has any effect on cancer and the US Federal Drugs Administration has obtained an injunction forbidding its distribution to patients.

Bibliography

Grossgebauer K 1995 The 'cancell' theory of carcinogenesis: re-evolution of an ancient, holistic neoplastic unicellular concept of cancer. Medical Hypotheses 45(6):545–555

## Cell specific cancer therapy

*Description*

This therapy is applied via a device which exposes the patient to a magnetic field, said to be weaker but more sensitive than magnetic resonance imaging (MRI). Treatment aims to detect and destroy active cancer cells without causing damage to healthy cells, thus enabling the body's immune system to work efficiently.

Evidence:   No supporting evidence could be found.

Safety:   No information regarding safety, contraindications or precautions was found.

Bibliography

No professional literature was found.

## Clark's 'cure for all cancers'

*Description*

This modality was devised by Hulda Clark, a naturopath, and is based on the theory that all cancers result from parasites, toxins and pollutants. A mixture of black walnut hulls, wormwood (*Artemisia absinthium*) and cloves (*Syzgium aromaticum*) are used to rid the body of over 100 parasites and claim to cure cancer in a just few days. Clark developed an electronic invention called a 'Syncrometer' which measures levels of 'ortho-phospho-tyrosine' levels in the patient to demonstrate the effectiveness of the remedy.

Evidence:   No clinical studies or other evidence could be found.

Safety:   Potentially serious central nervous system toxicity associated with wormwood and hepatotoxicity with walnuts could result from this treatment.

## Bibliography

No professional literature was found.

# Essiac

## Description

Essiac is a herbal remedy prescribed and promoted by Canadian nurse Rene Caisse. It contains burdock (*Arctium lappa/Arctium minus*), Indian rhubarb (*Rheum emodi Wall*), sheep sorrel (*Rumex acetosella*) and slippery elm (*Ulmus fulva*) and is said to be of Native American origin, legally available to cancer patients in Canada and widely used in North America.

Evidence:  Recent analyses of Essiac have demonstrated antioxidant and immune-modulatory properties and specific cytotoxicity relative to tumour growth. Significant CYP450 and inhibition of fibrinolysis were also shown. However, other studies have not demonstrated any real clinical value in using this remedy for the treatment of cancers, including breast cancer.

Safety:  No information regarding safety, contraindications or precautions was found. However one investigation appeared to demonstrate that essiac may stimulate the growth of breast cancer cells.

## Bibliography

Eberding A, Madera C, Xie S et al 2007 Evaluation of the antiproliferative effects of Essiac on in vitro and in vivo models of prostate cancer compared to paclitaxel. Nutrition and Cancer 58(2):188–196

Kaegi E 1998 Unconventional therapies for cancer: 1 Essiac. The task force on alternative therapies of the Canadian breast cancer research initiative. Canadian Medical Association Journal 158(7):897–902

Kulp K S, Montgomery J L, Nelson D O et al 2006 Essiac and Flor-Essence herbal tonics stimulate the in vitro growth of human breast cancer cells. Breast Cancer Research and Treatment 98(3):249–259

Ottenweller J, Putt K, Blumental E 2004 Inhibition of prostate cancer cell proliferation by Essiac. Journal of Alternative and Complementary Medicine 10(4):687–691

Leonard B J, Kennedy D A, Cheng F C et al 2006 An in vivo analysis of the herbal compound essiac. Anticancer Research 26(4B):3057–3063

Leonard S, Keil D, Mehiman T 2006 Essiac tea: scavenging of reactive oxygen species and effects on DNA damage. Journal of Ethnopharmacology 103(2):288–296

Seely D, Kennedy D A, Myers S P et al 2007 In vitro analysis of the herbal compound Essiac. Anticancer Research 27(6B):3875–3882

Tamayo C, Richardson M, Diamond S et al 2000 The chemistry and biological activity of herbs used in Flor-Essence herbal tonic and Essiac. Phytotherapy Research 14(1):1–14

Zick S, Sen A, Feng Y 2006 Trial of Essiac to ascertain its effects in women with breast cancer (TEA-BC). Journal of Alternative and Complementary Medicine 12(10):971–980

## Gerson diet

### Description

This is a detoxification diet used in the treatment of cancer and other degenerative conditions. An 8-week regimen involves extensive food preparation time, including the preparation of fresh juices as well as the ingestion of other additives, such as Lugol's solution (iodine and potassium iodide), thyroid extract and pancreatin and the use of coffee enemas, up to four times a day.

Evidence: No clinical trials were found which support the use of this intervention and there seems to be no evidence that it has any effect on cancer. Some of the references included here are very dated but give examples of information which is in the public domain.

Safety: Severe electrolyte imbalances and death can occur if taken to extremes. Not safe for children. Coffee enemas, in particular, which are also a component of other modalities for the treatment of cancer and some other life-limiting conditions, have been responsible for severe reactions, including death.

---

### Bibliography

Eisele J, Reay D 1980 Deaths related to coffee enemas. Journal of the American Medical Association 244(14):1608–1609

Green S 1992 A critique of the rationale for cancer treatment with coffee enemas and diet. Journal of the American Medical Association 268(22):3224–3227

Hildebrand F, Hildebrand L, Bradford K et al 1996 The role of follow-up and retrospective data analysis in alternative cancer management: the Gerson experience. Journal of Naturopathic Medicine 6(1):49–56

Hildenbrand G L, Hildenbrand L C, Bradford K et al 1995 Five-year survival rates of melanoma patients treated by diet therapy after the manner of Gerson: a retrospective review. Alternative Therapies in Health and Medicine 1(4):29–37

Molassiotis A, Peat P 2007 Surviving against all odds: analysis of 6 case studies of patients who followed the Gerson therapy. Integrative Cancer Therapies 6(1):80–88

Plaskett L 1998 Gerson therapy – a new approach. International Journal of Alternative and Complementary Medicine 16(1):9–14

### Resources

Gerson diet: www.Gersonsupportgroup.org.uk

## Grape cure

*Description*

The grape 'cure' was devised by Johanna Brandt who claimed that it helped to cure her stomach cancer, although there is now some doubt about her original diagnosis. The diet involves consumption solely of grapes or grape juice every 2 hours for up to 2 months, followed by gradual introduction of other fruits, then a raw food diet.

Safety:   The fact that this dietary regimen is termed a 'cure' is likely to give false hope to vulnerable patients. The diet is deficient in most nutrients, leading to the possibility of severe electrolyte imbalances, cardiac arrhythmias, hypotension and other pathological effects. Side-effects include: nausea, headaches, mucus production, weakness and muscle catabolism.

Evidence:   One recent review explored the benefits of grape seeds and green tea as chemoprotective agents, particularly in relation to prostate cancer, but no clinical trials appear to have been undertaken.

### Bibliography

Katiyar S K 2006 Matrix metalloproteinases in cancer metastasis: molecular targets for prostate cancer prevention by green tea polyphenols and grape seed proanthocyanidins. Endocrine, Metabolic and Immune Disorders Drug Targets 6(1):17–24

## Greek cancer cure

*Description*

The Greek cancer cure was proposed by microbiologist Dr Hariton-Tzannis Alivizatjos who claimed to have developed a blood test which could diagnose and indicate the type, severity and location of tumours. A serum, containing niacin, is then injected intravenously daily for up to 30 days and is said to stimulate the patient's immune system to destroy cancer cells and Alivizatjos claimed to have treated successfully numerous people with various types of cancer, including skin, bone, uterus, stomach and lymphatic system.

Evidence:   None found.

Safety:   The intravenous serum may contain levels of nicotinic acid in proportions high enough to cause burning at the injection site or erythema of the face and chest.

---

### Bibliography

No professional literature found.

## Hoxsey herbal treatment

*Description*

This treatment, developed by Harry Hoxsey during the 1920s and 1930s to treat internal and external cancers, involves the use of a collection of remedies derived from Native American medicine. External remedies include a red paste containing antimony trisulfide, zinc chloride, bloodroot, sulphur, an arsenic-containing powder and talcum powder. Internal remedies designed to re-balance the body's fluids consists of liquorice, burdock root, barberry, prickly ash, buckthorn bark, stillingia root and cascara plus other variations which have not been identified in the public arena. Patients receiving treatment are requested to refrain from eating tomatoes, vinegar, pork, alcohol, salt, sugar and white flour products, which are thought to affect the success of the remedies.

Evidence:   There is a limited amount of literature suggesting that the herbal paste may have a place in the treatment of some skin cancers. However, no clinical trials appear to have been published on either the efficacy or safety of this combination of herbal remedies, although there are several studies on the individual herbal components (see Herbal Medicine section).

Safety:   No information regarding safety was found. External remedies can be corrosive and destroy body tissue on contact.

Individual internal herbal medicines have specific contraindications and precautions.

Bibliography

Jellinek N, Maloney M E 2005 Escharotic and other botanical agents for the treatment of skin cancer: a review. Journal of the American Acadamy of Dermatology 53(3):487–495

## Hydrazine sulphate

*Description*

This treatment using hydrazine sulphate, devised during the 1970s to counteract the progressive weight loss of advanced cancer, is also claimed to cause tumour regression.

Evidence:   No clinical trials support the use of this intervention and there is no evidence that it has any effect on cancer.

Safety:   There is some evidence that hydrazine sulphate may cause nerve damage, hepatic and renal failure. Less life-threatening effects include nausea and vomiting, insomnia and hypoglycaemia.

Bibliography

Kaegi E 1998 Unconventional therapies for cancer: 4. Hydrazine sulphate. The task force on alternative therapies of the Canadian breast cancer research initiative. Canadian Medical Association Journal 158(10):1327–1330

Vickers A 2004 Alternative cancer cures: 'unproven' or 'disproven'? CA: a Cancer Journal for Clinicians 54(2):110–118

## Issels' treatment

*Description*

This treatment, devised by Dr Josef Issels (1907–1998), a pioneer in the immunological and microbiological approach to cancer, is based on the concept that malignant tumours do not develop in a healthy body with intact defences and good repair functions, that cancer is a systemic disease and that a tumour only becomes evident in the late stages of the disease. It consists of fever therapy, anti-cancer vaccines, a low protein, raw food diet, detoxification, removal of septic foci, homeopathic remedies and psychotherapy.

Evidence:    There is no evidence regarding the long-term outcomes for this treatment approach.

Safety:    No information regarding safety, contraindications or precautions was found.

### Bibliography

Issels R D 2006 High-risk soft tissue sarcoma: clinical trial and hyperthermia combined chemotherapy. International Journal of Hyperthermia 22(3): 235–239

Issels R D, Schlemmer M, Lindner L H 2006 The role of hyperthermia in combined treatment in the management of soft tissue sarcoma. Current Oncology Reports 8(4):305–309

### Resources

Issels Medical Centre: www.isselsmedicalcenter.com

## Kelley metabolic therapy

*Description*

This therapy, devised by William Kelley in the 1960s, is based on the premise that the development of tumours indicates a deficiency of pancreatic enzymes necessary to destroy cancer cells. Treatment consists of identification of the person's cancer index via a questionnaire, followed by detoxification with diuretics, colonic irrigation, deep breathing exercises, coffee enemas and sitz baths. This is combined with a restrictive diet, dependent on the person's metabolic type, involving ingestion of large quantities of daily supplements including digestive enzymes, animal glands and vitamins.

Evidence:    No supporting evidence was found.

Safety:    Electrolyte imbalance or vitamin toxicity resulting in death may occur. One out-of-date reference reports deaths occurring from the use of coffee enemas.

### Bibliography

Eisele J, Reay D 1980 Deaths related to coffee enemas. Journal of the American Medical Association 244(14):1608–1609

## Laetrile

*Description*

Laetrile is a combination of substances extracted from various plants, including the kernels of peaches, apricots, bitter almonds and other stone fruits and nuts. It was originally publicized as being able to control cancer, rather than cure it, claiming that it selectively killed the cancer cells. It is now used in conjunction with metabolic therapy.

Evidence:   No clinical trials are available which suggest that it has any effect on cancer.

Safety: Cyanide poisoning may occur from the chemical constituents of the various fruits and nuts. It should not be used in people with nut allergies.

**Bibliography**

Bromley J, Hughes-Brett G, Leong D et al 2005 Life threatening interaction between complementary medicine: cyanide toxicity following ingestion of amygdalin and vitamin C. Annals of Pharmacotherapy 39(9):1566–1569

Bromley J, Hughes-Brett G, Leong D et al 2005 Life threatening interaction between complementary medicine: cyanide toxicity following ingestion of amygdalin and vitamin C. Annals of Pharmacotherapy 39(9):1566–1569

Milazzo S, Lejeune S, Ernst E 2007 Laetrile for cancer: a systematic review of the clinical evidence. Supportive Care in Cancer 15(6):583–595

Vickers A 2004 Alternative cancer cures: unproven or disproven? CA: a Cancer Journal for Clinicians 54(2):110–118

## Livingstone-Wheeler regimen

*Description*

This regimen was devised by Dr Virginia Livingstone-Wheeler and is based on the theory that cancer is caused by a bacterium, which she called *Progenitor cryptocides* (later identified as *Staphylococcus epidermidis* a common skin bacterium), which invades the body when stressed. Treatment focuses on detoxification with a vegetarian diet, coffee enemas, blood transfusions, splenic extract, autologous vaccine prepared from the patient's own blood, antibiotics, vitamin and mineral supplementation, visualization and stress reduction.

Evidence:   No supporting evidence, either formal studies or reviews, could be found.

Safety:    In uncontrolled circumstances, severe electrolyte imbalances and death can occur.

Bibliography

No professional literature found.

## Metabolic therapy

*Description*

This therapy works on the theory that degenerative diseases such as cancer, multiple sclerosis and arthritis are caused by a metabolic imbalance due to accumulation of 'toxins' and includes a 'natural food' diet, coffee enemas, vitamins, minerals, glandular extracts, enzymes or laetrile.

Evidence:    No supporting evidence was found.

Safety:    In uncontrolled circumstances, severe electrolyte imbalances and death can occur due to nutritional deficiencies and the use of coffee enemas.

Bibliography

No professional literature was found.

## Mixed bacterial vaccines

*Description*

This therapy (formerly known as Coley toxins) is a treatment developed in the late 19th century by New York surgeon William Coley, a pioneer in immunotherapy. It involves injections of a mixture of killed cultures of *Streptococcus pyogenes* and *Serratia marcescens* to induce fever, which is thought to act as an immunostimulant in the treatment of cancer.

Evidence:    No clinical trials support the use of this intervention and there is no evidence that it has any effect on cancer.

Safety:    No information regarding safety, contraindications or precautions was found.

Bibliography

Richardson M, Ramirez T, Russell N 1999 Coley toxins immunotherapy: a retrospective review. Alternative Therapies in Health and Medicine 5(3):42–47

# Shark cartilage

*Description*

Shark cartilage is obtained from the spiny dogfish shark (*Squalus acanthias*) and the hammerhead shark (*Sphyrna lewini*). It is based on the incorrect assumption that sharks do not develop cancer and therefore have an inbuilt 'cure' for the disease by inhibiting blood vessel formation thus preventing tumour growth. Other claims for shark cartilage have focused on its purported wound healing and antiinflammatory effects. The active constituent is thought to be glycoproteins sphyrnastatin 1 and 2.

Evidence: There is some emerging evidence of possible effects of shark cartilage on the blood supply, preventing tumour growth.

Safety: Shark cartilage may cause hepatitis or lead to lowered blood sugar. Cartilage contains high levels of calcium, therefore it should not be used by people on calcium supplements or drugs which increase blood calcium levels.

### Bibliography

Ashar B, Vargo E 1996 Shark cartilage induced hepatitis. Annals of Internal Medicine 125:780–781

Bargahi A, Rabbani-Chadegani A 2008 Angiogenic inhibitor protein fractions derived from shark cartilage. Bioscience Reports 28(1):15–21

Batist G, Patenaude F, Champagne P et al 2002 Neovastat (AE-941 Shark cartilage) in refractory renal cell carcinoma patients: report of a phase 11 trial with two dose levels. Annals of Oncology 13(8):1259–1263

Bukowski R 2003 AE-941 A multifunctional anti-angiogenic compound: trials in renal cell carcinoma. Expert Opinion on Investigational Drugs 12(8):1403–1411

Dupont E, Falardeau P, Mousa S et al 2002 Anti-angiogenic and anti-metastatic properties of Neovastat (AE-941) an orally active extract from cartilage tissue. Clinical and Experimental Metastasis 19(2):145–153

Escudier B, Choueiri T K, Oudard S et al 2007 Prognostic factors of metastatic renal cell carcinoma after failure of immunotherapy: new paradigm from a large phase III trial with shark cartilage extract A E 941. Journal of Urology 178(5):1901–1905

Hammerness P, Barrette E, Szapary P 2002 Shark cartilage monograph: a clinical decision support tool. Journal of Herbal Pharmacotherapy 2(2):71–93

Jiagannath S, Champagne P, Hariton C et al 2003 Neovastat in multiple myeloma. European Journal of Haematology 70(4):267–268

Langman R, Walsh D 2003 Dangerous nutrition? Calcium, vitamin D and shark cartilage nutritional supplements and cancer related hypercalcemia. Supportive Care in Cancer 11(4):232–235

Loprinzi C, Levitt R, Barton D et al 2005 Evaluation of shark cartilage in patients with advanced cancer. Cancer 104(1):176–182

Mansberg G 2006 Cancer. Journal of Complementary Medicine 5(3):18–25

## Static electromagnetic field therapy

*Description*

This energy medicine is a form of electromagnetic therapy in which magnets are used to create a static electromagnetic field (as opposed to electromagnets which create an electromagnetic pulse). Its use in the treatment of cancer is based on the beliefs of the physician, William Philpott, that cancer is caused solely by acid hypoxia. Use of the static bio-north magnetic field enables an alkaline hyperoxia to be created, which is claimed to kill cancer cells. The bio-north magnet is placed over the cancerous lesion and kept in place for 3 months and the person is advised to use a magnetic chair with the flexible magnet placed over the heart during the day and to sleep on a magnetic mattress with a flexible magnet placed over the face. This programme is used in conjunction with a 4-day rotation diet and the avoidance of alcohol and tobacco.

Evidence: Static electromagnetic field therapy does not appear to increase the toxicity of concomitant chemotherapy.

Safety: The therapy appears, from recent work, to be relatively non-toxic, but no information regarding safety, precautions or contraindications was found.

Bibliography

Salvatore J R, Harrington J, Kummet T 2003 Phase I clinical study of a static magnetic field combined with anti-neoplastic chemotherapy in the treatment of human malignancy: initial safety and toxicity data. Bioelectromagnetics 24(7):524–527

## 714-X (Trimethylaminohydroxybicycloheptane chloride)

*Description*

This remedy was developed by the Canadian scientist and researcher, Gaston Naessens, who devised a microscope (somatoscope) with which he claimed to be able to identify live pathogens in blood which were distinct from bacteria and viruses. He termed these 'samatids' and suggested that they are present in people with serious illness, including cancer. By monitoring the lifecycle of these organisms he claimed to be able to map the disease process. The remedy, 714-X, which contains camphor, nitrogen, ammonium salts, sodium chloride and ethanol, was intended to disrupt the samatidian cycle. It was claimed to be more successful in people who had not received chemo- or radiotherapy and is thought to be useful prior to surgery to limit the spread of a tumour when incised during the operation.

Evidence: There are no clinical trials to support the use of this remedy and no evidence that it has any beneficial effect on cancer. Some animal studies have been conducted but have not shown 714-X to be effective in treating tumours.

Safety: No information regarding safety, contraindications or precautions was found. Mild side-effects have been reported including influenza-like symptoms and effects similar to those occurring during detoxification, including nausea, tiredness, headaches and low-grade fever.

Bibliography

Anonymous 1997 Court confirms conviction for peddling phony AIDS cure. AIDS Policy and Law 12(13):15

Kaegi E 1998 Unconventional therapies for cancer: 6. 714-X. Task force on alternative therapeutics of the Canadian breast cancer research initiative. Canadian Medical Association Journal, 158(12):1621–1624

# D

## Diagnostic techniques

*Description*

Various techniques are loosely included under the umbrella of complementary 'therapies', which are not generally therapeutic interventions, i.e. treatment, but rather alternative methods of reaching a diagnosis in order to plan treatment using other therapy modalities. In the House of Lords classification of complementary and alternative therapies (2000), diagnostic techniques constitute group 3b, having very little, if any, scientific basis.

Evidence: There is very little clinical literature available and no evidence in the form of appropriate scientific trials was found.

Safety: The principle safety issue is the delay in seeking appropriate medical diagnosis and treatment.

### Bibliography

Ernst E, Hentschel C 1995 Diagnostic methods in complementary medicine. Which craft is witchcraft? International Journal of Risk and Safety Medicine 7:55–63

Grace S, Vemulpad S, Beirman R 2006 Training in and use of diagnostic techniques among CAM practitioners: an Australian study. Journal of Alternative and Complementary Medicine 12(7):695–700

House of Lords Select Committee on Science and Technology 2000 Sixth report on complementary and alternative medicine. HMSO, London

## Dowsing

*Description*

Dowsing involves suspension of a pendulum over a person or specific body part, followed by interpretation of the movements made by the swinging pendulum, similar in principle to that of water divining. Medical dowsing is called radiesthesia and uses pendula and other instruments to focus psychic powers to aid diagnosis and selection of appropriate treatments, most commonly homeopathic remedies. Some people use dowsing as a way of life to help them avoid potentially harmful substances, such as nutrients to which they may be intolerant.

Evidence: There is no evidence to support this method of diagnosis.

Safety:   No specific safety issues have been identified.

Bibliography

Kapke K 2005 Energy medicine: radiesthesia: medical dowsing. Massage and Bodywork 20(3):122–126

McCarney R, Fisher P, Spink F et al 2002 Can homeopaths detect homeopathic medicines by dowsing? A randomized, double-blind, placebo-controlled trial. Journal of the Royal Society of Medicine 95(4):189–191

Vermeir K 2005 The 'physical prophet' and the powers of the imagination. Part II: a case-study on dowsing and the naturalisation of the moral, 1685–1710. Studies in History and Philosophy of Biological and Biomedical Sciences 36(1):1–24

Wegner D M 2004 Précis of the illusion of conscious will. Behavioral and Brain Sciences 27(5):649–659

Resources

British Society of Dowsers: www.britishdowsers.org

# Dynomizer

*Description*

This diagnostic technique was devised by the founder of radionics, Albert Abrams (1863–1924). It is based on his theory that electrons are the basic element of life and he developed a machine to measure the patient's electronic emissions, usually by analysing hair or blood. Interpretation of the corresponding vibrations enables a diagnosis to be made.

Evidence:   There is no evidence to support this method of diagnosis.

Safety:   No specific safety information was found.

Bibliography

No professional literature was found.

# Elimination diet

*Description*

An elimination diet is used to detect suspected food allergens which lead to intolerances and sensitivities which can trigger various health problems. A totally bland diet is eaten for up to 1 week in order to eliminate any foods which may cause adverse symptoms. Individual foods are then reintroduced singly to facilitate identification of any noticeable reactions.

Evidence:    No randomized controlled studies appear to have been undertaken on the effectiveness of elimination diets. The only professional literature found appears to debate the potential health issues related to unsupervised elimination diets, particularly where parents have attempted to treat children's allergies and intolerances to food.

Safety:    This diet should only to be undertaken under direct medical supervision as dietary deficiencies may manifest and anaphylaxis can occur following allergen challenge. It should not be used to aid diagnosis in children, pregnant women or the elderly and infirm unless specifically advocated by a doctor, as it may cause serious nutritional deficiencies which will impact on health and well-being.

### Bibliography

Drisko J, Bischoff B, Hall M et al 2006 Treating irritable bowel syndrome with a food elimination diet followed by food challenge and probiotics. Journal of the American College of Nutrition 25(6):514–522

Heyan M B; Committee on Nutrition 2006 Lactose intolerance in infants, children and adolescents. Pediatrics 118(3):1279–1286

Laitinen K, Isolauri E 2007 Allergic infants: growth and implications while on exclusion diets. Nestlé Nutrition Workshop Series. Paediatric Programme 60:157–169

Noimark L, Cox H E 2008 Nutritional problems related to food allergy in childhood. Pediatric Allergy and Immunology 19(2):188–195

Vlieg-Boerstra B J, van der Heide S, Bijleveld C M et al 2006 Dietary assessment in children adhering to a food allergen avoidance diet for allergy prevention. European Journal of Clinical Nutrition 60(12):1384–1390

### Resources

British Dietetic Association: www.bda.uk.com

## Face diagnosis

*Description*

This technique is used in naturopathy and is similar in principle to reflexology – in this case facial zones represent different regions and organs of the body. It has its roots in Ayurvedic, traditional Chinese and Japanese medicine.

Evidence:   There is no evidence to support this method of diagnosis.
Safety:   No specific safety information was found.

### Bibliography

No professional literature was found.

## Hair analysis

*Description*

Hair analysis is used by naturopaths, nutritional therapists and other practitioners as an aid to diagnosis. It enables identification of excess or deficient levels of trace metals from a sample of hair root, which is thought to reflect nutrients which have been ingested over the previous 3 months; the hair sample is burnt to ash which is then analysed for essential minerals.

Evidence:   There is no evidence to support this method of diagnosis, although it has been used by some authorities assisting couples planning to conceive, in the belief that it identifies nutritional deficiencies or inconsistencies which affect fertility.

Safety:   No specific safety information was found.

### Bibliography

Ernst E, Hentschel C 1995 Diagnostic methods in complementary medicine. Which craft is witchcraft? International Journal of Risk and Safety in Medicine 7:55–63

Niggemann B, Grüber C 2004 Unproven diagnostic procedures in IgE-mediated allergic diseases. Allergy 59(8):806–808

Passalacqua G, Compalati E, Schiappoli M et al 2005 Complementary and alternative medicine for the treatment and diagnosis of asthma and allergic diseases. Monaldi Archives for Chest Disease 63(1):47–54

## Iridology/iridiagnostics

*Description*

Iridology was developed by the Hungarian physician Ignatz von Peczely and involves close examination of the irises of the eyes. Abnormal appearance of the irises, such as flecks, discoloration, pressure signs and shape, are said to indicate potentially abnormal pathology. The principle is similar to that of reflexology in which a small part of the body represents a map of the whole. Far Eastern practitioners are beginning to use computer-assisted iridiagnosis.

Evidence:    A German study investigated the accuracy of iridology in diagnosing colorectal cancer, but the results were statistically no better than chance. Others have explored its value in detecting hypertension.

Safety:    No specific safety information was found.

## Bibliography

Cho J J, Hwang W J, Hong S H et al 2008 Angiotensinogen gene polymorphism predicts hypertension and iridological constitutional classification enhances the risk for hypertension in Koreans. International Journal of Neuroscience 118(5):635–645

Ernst E 2000 Iridology: not useful and potentially harmful. Archives of Ophthalmology 118(1):120–121

Herber S, Rehbein M, Tepas T et al 2008 [Looking for colorectal cancer in the patients iris?] Ophthalmologie 105(6):570–574

He J F, Ye H N, Ye M Y 2002 [The automatic iris map overlap technology in computer-aided iridiagnosis.] Zhongguo Yi Liao Qi Xie Za Zhi 26(6):395–397

Münstedt K, El-Safadi S, Brück F 2005 Can iridology detect susceptibility to cancer? A prospective case-controlled study. Journal of Alternative and Complementary Medicine 11(3):515–519

Niggemann B, Grüber C 2004 Unproven diagnostic procedures in IgE mediated allergic diseases. Allergy 59(8):806–808

Passalacqua G, Compalati E, Schiappoli M et al 2005 Complementary and alternative medicine for the treatment and diagnosis of asthma and allergic diseases. Monaldi Archives for Chest Diseases 63(1):47–54

Um J Y, An N H, Yang G B et al 2005 Novel approach of molecular genetic understanding of iridology: relationship between iris constitution and angiotensin converting enzyme gene polymorphism. American Journal of Chinese Medicine 33(3):501–505

Yoo C S, Hwang W J, Hong S H et al 2007 Relationship between iris constitution analysis and TNF-alpha gene polymorphism in hypertensives. American Journal of Chinese Medicine 35(4):621–629

## Resources

Guild of Naturopathic Iridologists: www.gni-international.org

# Kinesiology

*Description*

This is based on the theory that a feedback loop exists between the body's inner organs and the muscles, particularly in the upper arm, biceps and quadriceps. If an organ fails to function properly or as a reaction to injury or stress, toxins accumulate around the related muscle, causing weakness. Kinesiologists test the strength of various muscle groups using the principles of traditional Chinese medicine to determine which body systems are out of balance. It is often used to test for allergies and food intolerances. Touch for Health is a simplified form of kinesiology and involves testing of 42 muscles to determine energy imbalances of the meridian system which can then be treated with acupressure. There is a significant difference in attitudes to kinesiology between the UK and the North Americas, with postgraduate degrees in the subject being available in some US and Canadian universities.

Evidence:    There is some emerging evidence, primarily from the USA and Canada, but also from some European countries, that kinesiology may be effective in detecting physiological variations which may contribute to a full diagnosis in conjunction with conventional investigations.

Safety:    No specific safety information was found.

### Bibliography

Hall S, Lewith G, Brien S et al 2008 A review of the literature in applied and specialised kinesiology. Forschende Komplementärmedizin 15(1):40–46

Hansen S, Tremblay L, Elliott D 2008 Real-time manipulation of visual displacement during manual aiming. Human Movement Science 27(1):1–11

Niggemann B, Grüber C 2004 Unproven diagnostic procedures in IgE-mediated allergic diseases. Allergy 59(8):806–808

Passalacqua G, Compalati E, Schiappoli M et al 2005 Complementary and alternative medicine for the treatment and diagnosis of asthma and allergic diseases. Monaldi Archives for Chest Diseases 63(1):47–54

Waxenegger I, Endler P C, Wulkersdorfer B et al 2007 Individual prognosis regarding effectiveness of a therapeutic intervention using pre-therapeutic 'kinesiology muscle test'. Scientific World Journal 7:1703–1707

### Resources

Association of Systematic Kinesiology: www.kinesiology.co.uk

# Kirlian photography

*Description*

This technique involves photographing the low level electromagnetic energy field around the human body (sometimes referred to as the aura), thought to be detectable as barely visible light (bio-photoemissions). It is used to detect alterations of shape and colour which may indicate changes in emotional state, energy and health. The person is placed within a high-frequency, alternating electric field which interacts with his/her electromagnetic energy field. A photographic representation can then be interpreted and a possible diagnosis made.

Evidence:    One study has explored the variations between different gemstones, as depicted with Kirlian photography.

Safety:    No specific safety information was found.

---

### Bibliography

---

Duerden T 2004 An aura of confusion Part 2: the aided eye – 'imaging the aura'? Complementary Therapies in Nursing and Midwifery 10(2):116–123

Vainshelboim A, Momoh K S 2005 Bioelectrographic testing of mineral samples: a comparison of techniques. Journal of Alternative and Complementary Medicine 11(2):299–304

---

### Resources

---

Kirlian Research Ltd: www.kirlian.co.uk

## Radionics

*Description*

Developed by Albert Abrams (1863–1924), radionics is based on the concept that diseased tissue radiates abnormal wave patterns which adversely influence a healthy person, causing illness. It is thought that human energy is transmitted through material objects which can be 'read' by the activation of a 'black box'; diagnosis is claimed to be possible irrespective of the presence or otherwise of the patient. Diagnosis is made from a medical questionnaire and a 'witness' – usually a sample of hair or blood – placed in the black box which is tuned to the vibrational levels of a range of diseases. Treatment encompasses the healing energy from an appropriate remedy (homeopathic or herbal).

Evidence:    There is no evidence to support this method of diagnosis.

Safety:    No specific safety information was found.

Bibliography

No professional literature was found.

Resources

Radionics Association: www.radionic.co.uk

## Skull diagnosis

*Description*

This method involves palpation of various areas of the skull which are associated with certain muscles, to facilitate recognition of imbalance in these muscles. Treatment incorporates gentle stretching of the relevant area of the scalp followed by local treatment of the identified muscle.

Evidence:    There is no evidence to support this method of diagnosis.

Safety:    No specific safety information was found.

Bibliography

No professional literature was found.

## Temple diagnosis

*Description*

In this technique, used in naturopathy, trigger points on the tempero-sphenoidal line are palpated to diagnose sources of pain or to detect imbalances in the spinal column or an over-riding muscle.

Evidence:    No evidence was found.

Safety:    No specific safety information was found.

Bibliography

No professional literature was found.

## Vega test

*Description*

The Vega test purports to measure resistance to the flow of electricity over acupuncture points at the ends of the fingers and toes. The process involves application of homeopathic dilutions of various substances, including allergens, bacteria, viruses or diseased tissue; the Vega machine detects reactions to each substance and the information is then interpreted to identify the causes of the person's ill-health.

Evidence:   Although some studies have demonstrated that the Vega test may detect food intolerances, it does not appear to be 100% successful.

Safety:   No specific safety information was available.

### Bibliography

Herman P M, Drost L M 2004 Evaluating the clinical relevance of food sensitivity tests: a single subject experiment. Alternative Medical Review 9(2):198–207

Lewith G, Kenyon J, Broomfield J et al 2001 The vega test has no reliability or validity in diagnosing allergies. British Medical Journal 322:131–134

## Energy medicine/energy field medicine

*Description*

Energy – or vibrational – medicine is based on the concept that each individual has not only a physical and biochemical basis, but also a complex system of energy which facilitates homeostasis and which is subsidiary to the earth's universal energy field. It is thought that the human body has six dynamic energy systems flowing through and around it, variously termed 'life-force', 'aura', 'vital force' (homeopathy), prana (Ayurvedic medicine), Qi (Chinese medicine) or Ki (Japanese medicine). There are six energy systems: acoustic, thermal, elastic, electromagnetic, photonic and gravitational energy. It is believed that disturbances in the individual's energy field, either from internal sources such as trauma, stored emotions, negative thoughts and actions or from external sources, including infective organisms and environmental factors result in lowered vitality leading to disease of the body, mind or spirit. During treatment, the practitioner's and patient's energy fields are connected by a two-way energy exchange which forms an energy or auric field, which is then focused therapeutically to promote wellness and healing.

The aura is the electromagnetic energy field (also known as the bioenergetic coronal discharge), which is believed to surround the human body. It is generally invisible to the naked eye, but is claimed to be visible to particularly sensitive people. Kirlian photography purports to produce a visual photographic representation of the aura. There are seven auric field layers: the etheric body, which is closest to the material body; the emotional and mental bodies; the astral body, transcending matter and spirit; the causal body focusing on life purpose; the celestial body influencing insight, inspiration and clairvoyance; and the spiritual or cosmic consciousness, which is in direct contact with the divine universe.

*Note*: Certain forms of energy medicine are not included here but are covered in other relevant sections.

Evidence:  Some tentative evidence is emerging, although none is based on randomized controlled trials.

Safety: No information regarding safety, contraindications or precautions was found.

### Bibliography

Engebretson J, Wardell D W 2007 Energy based modalities. Nursing Clinics of North America 42(2):243–259

Gulmen F 2004 Energy medicine. American Journal Chinese Medicine 32(5): 651–658

Hankey A 2004 Are we close to a theory of energy medicine? Journal of Alternative and Complementary Medicine 10(1):83–86

Osborn K 2005 Energy medicine: a field of potential. Massage and Bodywork 20(4):16–26

Wootton J 2004 Energy medicine: information and research resources on the web. Journal of Alternative and Complementary Medicine 10(1):183–185

Young G, Smith S, Avanozian V et al 2004 Biofield perception: a series of pilot studies with cultured human cells. Journal of Alternative and Complementary Medicine 10(3):463–467

## Absent/distant/psi healing

*Description*

This technique was devised by the spiritual healer, Harry Edwards. It focuses on freeing the mind from distraction, facilitating receptiveness to healing energies, mental communication with the affected person and relaxation and visualization and involves intercession by a healer on behalf of the person, who may not necessarily be present at the time. It may include prayer and/or visualization of the transfer of healing energy towards the person, often using appropriate colours and then visualizing the person as being free from disease and 'whole'.

Evidence: There is some evidence that this intervention offers palliative care and psychological support, improving quality of life, particularly in those with life-limiting illness.

Safety: No information regarding safety, contraindications or precautions was found.

### Bibliography

Astin J, Stone J, Abrams D et al 2006 The efficacy of distant healing for human immunodeficiency virus: results of a randomised trial. Alternative Therapies in Health and Medicine 12(6):36–41

Crawford C, Sparber A, Jonas W 2003 A systematic review of the quality of research on hands-on and distance healing: clinical and laboratory studies. Alternative Therapies in Health and Medicine 9(3 Suppl):A96–A104

Ebneter M, Binder M, Saller R 2001 Distant healing and clinical research. Forschende Komplementärmedizin und Klassische Naturheilkunde 8(5):274–287

Schiltz M, Radin D, Malle B et al 2003 Distant healing intention: definitions and evolving guidelines for laboratory studies. Alternative Therapies in Health and Medicine 9(3 Suppl):A31–A43

### Resources

National Federation of Spiritual Healers: www.nfsh.org.uk/distanthealing

## Bio-electromagnetic therapy/magnetic field therapy/ electromagnetic therapy

*Description*

Bio-electromagnetics is the study of the interaction of living organisms with electromagnetic fields, based on the notion that all living organisms have a bio-electromagnetic foundation which is influenced by external electromagnetic emissions from the earth's geomagnetic field. Harmful rays emanating from the earth cause geopathic stress (disease of the earth) which can cause physical, emotional or spiritual ill-health to humans. This may happen naturally when the earth's radiation is distorted by weak electromagnetic fields caused by subterranean running water, mineral concentrations, fault lines or underground cavities or may be man-made, such as emanations from electricity power lines interrupting geopathic stress lines. Other modern-day causes include televisions, visual display units, microwave ovens and mobile telephones. Therapy involves the use of bio-magnetic poles, the magnet's North Pole being negatively charged and likened to the concept of Yin in Traditional Chinese Medicine and used for detoxifying, clearing and cooling. The magnet's South Pole is positively charged, corresponds to the concept of Yang in Chinese medicine and is used for heating, stimulating and accumulating effects. The aim of treatment is to restore the person's electromagnetic balance.

Evidence:   There is some evidence that this intervention can provide pain relief in certain conditions, notably neuromusculoskeletal conditions.

Safety: This intervention is contraindicated for people fitted with pacemakers or internal defibrillators.

### Bibliography

Langford J, McCarthy P 2005 Randomised controlled clinical trial of magnet use in chronic low back pain: a pilot study. Clinical Chiropractic 8(1):13–19

Laser T 2003 Magnetic therapy – quackery or a new dimension in medicine? An overview. Krankengymnastik 55(6):970–974

Weintraub M, Cole S 2004 Pulsed magnetic file therapy in refractory neuropathic pain secondary to peripheral neuropathy: electro diagnostic parameters pilot study. Neurorehabilitation and Neural Repair 18(1):42–46

Weintraub M, Cole S 2005 Pulsed magnetic field therapy in refractory carpal tunnel syndrome: electro diagnostic parameters pilot study. Journal of Back and Musculoskeletal Rehabilitation 18(3–4):79–83

Weintraub M, Wolfe G, Barohn R et al 2003 Static magnetic field therapy for symptomatic diabetic retinopathy: a randomised, double-blind, placebo-controlled trial. Archives of Physical Medicine and Rehabilitation 84(5):736–746

## Colour therapy

### Description

This therapy has its roots in antiquity when colour and light were used to treat disease and healing temples were painted in specific colours. In Ayurvedic medicine, colours are considered to have particular properties, e.g. red is stimulating and warming, while silver is cooling. Modern colour therapy works on the principle that certain organs and systems of the body respond to the frequency, wavelength and energy of specific colour treatments applied to different parts of the body; the colours correcting physical and mental vibrational imbalances. For example, blue is used to treat insomnia; pink to reduce aggression; green for nervous tension. Therapy may be directed at the chakras of the body, a component of Ayurvedic and other traditional medicine systems. Treatment will also include recommended colour choices of clothes, food and the person's environment. Aura-soma involves self-selection of four significant colours which are thought to represent the current physical and emotional state of the affected person; daily dermal application of these colours enables the body to absorb the colour in order for homeostasis to be restored. Colour-puncture is a derivative of acupuncture which directs selected coloured light onto acupuncture points in the belief that the skin is photosensitive, the colour therefore being absorbed into the skin and penetrating the body's cells.

Evidence: Some evidence supports the use of colour therapy in behaviour modification; consideration has been given to the most appropriate colour for phototherapy treatment of neonatal physiological jaundice.

Safety: No information regarding safety, contraindications or precautions was found.

### Bibliography

Croke M 2002 Introducing esogetic colorpuncture: a wholistic system of acu-light therapy for body, mind and soul. Beginnings 22(2):10–11

Deppe A 1999 Light relief: the case for ocular light therapy. Australian Journal of Holistic Nursing 6(2):42–44

Ebbesen F, Madsen P, Støvring S 2007 Therapeutic effect of turquoise versus blue light with equal irradiance in preterm infants with jaundice. Acta Paediatrica 96(6):837–841

Marsh D 1997 Seeing pink. International Journal of Alternative and Complementary Medicine 15(12):27–28

Rubaltelli F F 2007 Blue light, green light, turquoise light: do we need to change our devices to treat our jaundiced preterm infants? Acta Paediatrica 96(6):792–793

Steinberg H 2007 A new 'light' on color light therapy: visual color therapy and the effect on disease conditions. Townsend Letters 292:98–99

Strawn J 1999 The healing power of color. Alternative Health Practitioner 5(2):173–174

### Resources

International Association of Colour: www.internationalassociationofcolour.com
Aura Soma: www.bomi.info/practitioners/aurasoma

## Crystal/gem therapy

### Description

In this therapy, gems or crystals are used to detect and clear energy blockages and promote health and well-being. It is based on the theory that crystalline substances collect, focus and emit electromagnetic energy; in Ayurvedic medicine, crystals are particularly targeted to restore chakra balance. Different crystals are used for different conditions and are sometimes rendered down to a fine powder and combined with plant essences for particular treatments. Electro-crystal therapy, a later development by Harry Oldfield in 1988, employs a system of pulsed high-frequency currents and electromagnetic induction. Selected crystals are added to a saline solution, applied to the person's body and a current of electricity is passed through the solution to initiate healing. It is based on the belief that each of the body's tissues resonates to a specific frequency, which is altered by illness: healing is achieved by applying the appropriate frequency, via the gems, to the diseased area. The electro-frequencies most used in electro-crystal therapy are those emanated by the chakras, between 1 Hz and 45 kHz.

Evidence:   None was found.

Safety:   No information regarding safety, contraindications or precautions was found.

### Bibliography

No professional literature was found.

### Resources

Crystal healing: www.crystal-healing.org

## Environmental medicine/clinical ecology

*Description*

This therapy is based on the 1940s work of Theron Randolph and focuses on the effects of environmental factors such as pollution, environmental chemicals, electromagnetic radiation and geopathic stress on the human body. These are thought to cause abnormal behaviour, allergies, asthma, cancer, mood changes, reproductive dysfunction and neurological illnesses in susceptible people. The response to exposure to these factors depends on the person's susceptibility and can manifest differently from person to person, depending on genetics, nutritional status and effectiveness of detoxifying pathways. Treatment is determined after taking a careful history, with special attention to the home and work environment, followed by allergy testing, an elimination diet if appropriate or other diagnostic techniques and may include avoidance of the relevant toxins, desensitization and teaching the person specific techniques to cope with the problem.

Evidence:    None was found.

Safety:  No    information    regarding    safety,    contraindications    or precautions was found.

Bibliography

Vanelli M, Chiari G, Gugliotta M et al 2002 Diabetes and alternative medicine: diabetic patients' experiences with Ayur-Ved, 'clinical ecology' and 'cellular nutrition' methods. Minerva Pediatrica 54(2):165–169

## Faith/spiritual healing/therapeutic prayer

*Description*

This is a form of healing practised within a mainstream religion and may include a non-denominational energy exchange or channelling between healer and patient, with or without prayer intercession.

Evidence:    There is some evidence that this intervention alters pain perception. It may also improve quality of life in chronically or terminally ill people, but whether this is due to a placebo effect is unknown.

Safety:    No   information   regarding   safety   or   contraindications   was found. It should not be used in place of orthodox treatment.

Bibliography

Abbot N, Harkness C, Stevinson C et al 2001 Spiritual healing as a therapy for chronic pain: a randomised, clinical trial. Pain 91(1–2):79–89

Gerard S, Smith B, Simpson J 2003 A randomised controlled trial of spiritual healing in restricted back movement. Journal of Alternative and Complementary Medicine 9(4):467–477

Harkness E 2001 Quality of life in chronically ill patients treated by spiritual healing. Focus on Alternative and Complementary Therapies 6(3):210

Jonas W, Crawford C 2003 Science and spiritual healing: a critical review of spiritual healing 'energy medicine' and intentionality. Alternative Therapies in Health and Medicine 9(2):56–61

Taylor E 2005 Spiritual complementary therapies in cancer care. Seminars in Oncology Nursing 21(3):159–163

Wiesendager H, Werthmuller L, Reuter K et al 2001 Chronically ill patients treated by spiritual healing improve in quality of life: results of a randomised waiting list controlled study. Journal of Alternative and Complementary Medicine 7(1):45–51

Resources

National Federation of Spiritual Healers: www.nfsh.org.uk/distanthealing

## Healing touch/biotherapy

*Description*

Healing touch is actually a non-touch intervention developed by nurse, Janet Mentgen, and is an amalgam of her own energy-based techniques with those from other therapies such as Therapeutic Touch, Healing Science and Native American (Hopi Indian) traditions.

Evidence:   There is some evidence that healing touch offers palliative care and improves quality of life in chronically and terminally ill people. However, the term 'healing touch' can be used generically and not all references relate to the specific form of biotherapy.

Safety:   No information regarding safety or contraindications was found, however caution should be taken regarding using it in place of orthodox treatment.

Bibliography

Berden M, Jerman O, Skarja M 1997 A possible physical basis for healing touch (biotherapy) evaluated by high voltage electrophotography. Acupuncture and Electro-therapeutics Research 22(2):127–146

Engebretson J, Wind-Wardell D 2007 Energy based modalities. Nursing Clinics of North America 42(2):243–259

Maville J A, Bowen J E, Benham G 2008 Effect of healing touch on stress perception and biological correlates. Holistic Nursing Practice 22(2):103–110

Taylor B, Lo R 2001 The effects of healing touch on the coping ability, self esteem and general health of undergraduate nursing students. Complementary Therapies in Nursing and Midwifery 7(1):34–42

Wardell D, Rintala D, Duan Z et al 2006 A pilot study of healing touch and progressive relaxation for chronic neuropathic pain in persons with spinal chord injury. Journal of Holistic Nursing 24(4):231–240

Wilkinson D, Knox P, Chatman J et al 2002 The clinical effectiveness of healing touch. Journal of Alternative and Complementary Medicine 8(1):33–47

Wind-Wardell D 2000 The trauma release technique: how it is taught and experienced in healing touch. Alternative Complementary Therapies 6(1):20–27

Resources

Healing touch: www.healing-touch.co.uk

# Krieger–Kuntz method (formerly Therapeutic Touch)

*Description*

This technique was developed by Dr Delores Krieger and Dora van Kuntz and has long been incorporated into American nursing practice. It is based on the ancient concept of 'laying on of hands' and aims to re-balance and re-pattern the energy field surrounding the patient. The practitioner centres him/herself and focuses on the intention to heal. S/he moves the hands over the patient, noting any imbalances in the aura as identified by changes in temperature, pressure, rhythm or tingling sensation, then returns to these areas and uses a head-to-toe smoothing action (called unruffling) and re-patterns the disturbed energy field, bringing it back into harmony by intent and visualization.

Evidence: Several studies have investigated the potential pain-relieving effects of this method of healing; others have explored the psychological and neurological benefits, e.g. in anxiety and Alzheimer's disease.

Safety: No information regarding safety, contraindications or precautions was found.

### Bibliography

Coppa D 2008 The internal process of Therapeutic Touch. Journal of Holistic Nursing 26(1):17–24

Frank L S, Frank J L, March D et al 2007 Does Therapeutic Touch ease the discomfort or distress of patients undergoing stereotactic core breast biopsy? A randomized clinical trial. Pain Medicine 8(5):419–424

Hawranik P, Johnston P, Deatrich J 2008 Therapeutic Touch and agitation in individuals with Alzheimer's disease. Western Journal of Nursing Research 30(4):417–434

Huff M B, McClanahan K K, Omar H A 2006 From healing the whole person: an argument for Therapeutic Touch as a complement to traditional medical practice. Scientific World Journal 6:2188–2195

Jackson E, Kelley M, McNeil P et al 2008 Does Therapeutic Touch help reduce pain and anxiety in patients with cancer? Clinical Journal of Oncology Nursing 12(1):113–120

Robinson J, Biley F C, Dolk H 2007 Therapeutic Touch for anxiety disorders. Cochrane Database of Systematic Reviews (3):CD006240

### Resources

Nurse Healers Professional Association International: www.therapeutic-touch.org

## 'Laying on of hands'

*Description*

The concept of laying on of hands has been recorded since ancient times. There has been renewed interest in the area of energy medicine in recent years and the increased popularity of such therapies as reiki and the Krieger–Kunz method of Therapeutic Touch indicates its acceptance. Energy field disturbance is now a method of nursing diagnosis in America.

Evidence:   There is some evidence that this intervention offers palliative care and improves quality of life.

Safety:   No information regarding safety or contraindications was found, however caution if using in place of orthodox treatment.

Bibliography

Kelley M 2002 Strategies for innovative energy-based nursing practice: the Healing Touch program. SCI Nursing 19(3):117–124

Umbreit A W 2000 Healing touch: applications in the acute care setting. AACN Clinical Issues 11(1):105–119

## Neural therapy

*Description*

Neural therapy was founded by the German physician, Ferdinand Huneke, in 1940 and is based on his theory of interference fields, interruptions to the flow of electrical energy thought to be responsible for chronic illness. Injections of local anaesthetics are thought to destroy these interference fields, allowing healing to take place. Neural therapy is used for a wide range of conditions including allergies, chronic pain, asthma, reducing keloid scar tissue and skin disorders. Localities for injections include acupuncture points, scars, peripheral nerves, glands and trigger points.

Evidence:   None found.

Safety: No information regarding safety, contraindications or precautions was found.

Bibliography

No professional literature was found.

## Pattern therapy

*Description*

This therapy is based on the notion that geometric shapes exert power over our spiritual lives and can aid healing, a concept acknowledged by many ancient cultures which understood the importance of patterns or shapes, especially in buildings. Pattern therapy was developed by Dr A Westlake, who found that patterns can be a valuable aid to psionic medicine. The relevant remedy is placed in the centre of a three-dimensional pattern, shapes and forms being aesthetically pleasing and contributing to a healing environment. An example of this is anthroposophical clinics which are constructed with smooth rounded walls to provide a calm and relaxing atmosphere.

Evidence:    None was found.

Safety:   No information regarding safety, contraindications or precautions was found. However, it should be remembered that some pattern configurations may induce epilepsy.

### Bibliography

No professional literature was found.

## Polarity therapy

*Description*

Polarity therapy was developed by Randolph Stone (1890–1981), from a synthesis of Ayurvedic and traditional Chinese medicine. It consists of bodywork to facilitate reorganization of the person's energy fields (similar to Reiki) and exercise based on hatha yoga which aims to increase awareness of energy flow through the body. A vegetarian diet is advocated, with a predominance of raw food, harnessing the energetic component of food. Polarity tea, a combination of fennel, fenugreek, flax, liquorice and peppermint, is also prescribed. Counselling is incorporated into the treatment to allow the person to express and release feelings.

Evidence:    Some authorities have investigated the potential use of polarity therapy for people with dementia.

Safety: No information on safety, contraindications or precautions was found. There is however evidence of risks and contraindications of the individual herbs use in polarity tea, as well as the possible interactions with other herbs and with prescribed pharmacological preparations (see Herbal Medicine section).

### Bibliography

Anderson E 2001 Energy therapies for physical and occupational therapists working with older adults. Physical and Occupational Therapy in Geriatrics 18(4):35–49

Benford M, Tainagi J, Burr-Doss D et al 1999 Gamma radiation fluctuations during alternative healing therapy. Alternative Therapies in Health and Medicine 5(4):51–56

Korn L, Loytomaki S, Hinman T 2007 Polarity therapy protocol for dementia caregivers – part 2. Journal of Bodywork and Movement Therapies 11(3):244–259

Korn L, Ryser R 2007 Designing a polarity therapy protocol: bridging holistic, cultural and biomedical models of research. Journal of Bodywork and Movement Therapies 11(2):129–140

Megidesh L 2001 Polarity therapy: energy medicine to balance and heal the life-force. Alternative and Complementary Therapies 7(5):296–303

Oschman J 2002 Clinical aspects of biological fields: an introduction for healthcare professionals. Journal of Bodywork and Movement Therapies 6(2):117–125

Vanderbilt S 2005 The hidden patient: polarity therapy for dementia caregivers. Massage and Bodywork 20(6):78–86

### Resources

UK Polarity Therapy Association: www.ukpta.org.uk

## Psionic medicine

*Description*

This is a post-graduate branch of medicine, devised by Dr George Laurence, which integrates homeopathy, radiesthesia and orthodox medicine, utilizing paranormal faculties, including the use of 'witnesses' pendulums, colour, dowsing and radiesthetic techniques to determine the best treatment.

Evidence: None found.

Safety: No information regarding safety, contraindications or precautions was found.

Bibliography

No professional literature was found.

Resources

The Psionic Medical Society: www.psionicmedicine.org

## Sound therapy/auditory stimulation

*Description*

Sound therapy is based on the principle that everything on earth, including the human body, is in a state of constant auditory vibration. Certain sounds are thought to be therapeutic, harnessing both the auditory sound and the physical or vibrational effect. Each body tissue is thought to resonate at a specific frequency which is altered by illness; therapy consists of targeting of sound waves at an appropriate frequency onto specific areas of the body.

Music is the most commonly used form of sound therapy. In toning, the person relieves stress by forming elongated vowel sounds thought to resonate through the body, similar in concept to Gregorian chanting. Cymatic therapy uses computerized sound waves transmitted through the skin in a similar manner to acupuncture and is based on the theory that illness is caused by unbalanced resonance in the specific tissue, the use of the correct sound frequency helping to re-balance the tissues and promote healing. Infratonic QGM machine therapy uses sound frequencies to reduce pain and ease headaches and is thought to simulate the secondary sound waves emitted by Qigong masters. The Tomatis method simulates the stages of hearing development from intrauterine life to a baby's first sounds (called sonic birth) and re-patterns the hearing range and attention span. In cases of hearing loss, the ear is stimulated by listening at low volume to highly filtered classical music presenting alternating high and low tones. Auditory integration training, developed by French physician Guy Berard, is based on the belief that behavioural and cognitive disorders are due to distorted perception of sound frequencies; treatment involves the use of a device which desensitizes people who are hypersensitive to high frequency sounds.

Evidence: Some studies support the use of sound therapy in behaviour modification. Auditory stimulation has been used successfully to complement other alternative and conventional treatments to turn a breech-presenting fetus to cephalic. The Tomatis method has been used with autistic children and it may play a part in those with attention deficit disorder.

Safety: No information regarding safety, contraindications or precautions was found.

### Bibliography

Barber C 1999 The use of music and colour theory as a behaviour modifier. British Journal of Nursing 8(7):443–448

Baumgaertel A 1999 Alternative and controversial treatments for attention-deficit/hyperactivity disorder. Pediatric Clinics of North America 46(5):977–992

Brodie R 1999 Healing with sound and colour. Journal of Alternative and Complementary Therapies 17(3):19–21

Johnson R L, Elliott J P 1995 Fetal acoustic stimulation, an adjunct to external cephalic version: a blinded, randomized crossover study. American Journal of Obstetrics and Gynecology 173(5):1369–1372

Leeds J 1997 Therapeutic music and sound in healthcare Part 2: the Tomatis method-frequency medicine for the 21st century. American Journal of Acupuncture 25(4):299–305

Porcaro C, Zappasodi F, Barbati G et al 2006 Fetal auditory responses to external sounds and mother's heart beat: detection improved by Independent Component Analysis. Brain Research 1101(1):51–58

Sinha Y, Silove N, Wheeler D et al 2004 Auditory integration training and other sound therapies for autism spectrum disorders. Cochrane Database of Systematic Reviews(1):CD003681

Wauters A 2007 Homeopathic colour and sound remedies. Homeopath 26(2):57–59

Zucker M 2000 Healing with Vedic sounds East meets West on the quantum level. Townsend Letters 202:60–64

### Resources

The Listening Centre (Lewes), East Sussex: Tel 01273 474877

## Zero balancing

*Description*

Zero balancing was developed by an American doctor and osteopath in 1973, Dr Fritz Smith. It aims to restore energy flow throughout the body, particular attention being paid to weight-bearing joints, eyes and breathing patterns in order to balance deeper structures which are the conduits of the body's energy. Re-balanced energy flow is claimed to improved posture and to promote physical, mental and spiritual homeostasis.

Evidence:    None was found.

Safety: No information regarding safety, contraindications or precautions was found.

### Bibliography

Edmunds D, Gafner G 2003 Touching trauma: combining hypnotic ego strengthening and zero balancing. Contemporary Hypnosis 20(4):215–220

Geggus P 2004 Introduction to the concepts of zero balancing. Journal of Bodywork and Movement Therapies 8(1):58–71

Ralston A 1998 Zero balancing: information on a therapy. Complementary Therapies in Nursing Midwifery 4(2):41–46

### Resources

The Zero Balancing Association, UK: www.zerobalancinguk.org

# H

## Herbal medicine/medical herbalism/phytotherapy

*Description*

Herbal medicine is the study and use of plants as medicines or food nutrients to restore and maintain good health. Western medical herbalists follow similar diagnostic procedures as orthodox doctors including history-taking, laboratory tests and X-rays necessary, examination and prescription of appropriate remedies. Treatment may consist of four elements: cleansing, detoxification and elimination, with expectorants, laxatives and diuretics; heating and aiding circulation with circulatory stimulants, peripheral vasodilators and aromatic digestives; cooling with bitters to stimulate digestion and febrifuges to reduce temperature; and tonification to nourish and repair with tonic herbs, often combined with convalescence, rest, exercise and diet.

Herbal medicine is found in every society and is probably the oldest form of therapeutic intervention known to humankind. Practitioners, now known as medical herbalists, have also been called 'wise women', folk healers or herbista; in other cultures they may be known by a local term, e.g. Mexican curanderas/curanderos, traditional Chinese medicine practitioners or Ayurvedic doctors. Herbalists in England have been allowed to practise under the Herbalists' Charter awarded by King Henry VIII in 1542; modern practice is voluntarily regulated. Training is monitored, primarily, by the National Institute of Medical Herbalists which was founded in 1864. However, under the above Charter and English Common Law, anyone can practise as a herbalist without formal qualifications, although changes within European complementary medicine regulation may change this in the near future.

Herbal remedies (defined in (2004/27/EC Article 1) are subject to the EU Traditional and Herbal Medicines Directive (2004/24/EC) and Medicinal Products for Human Use (2004/27/EC). The key difference between herbal remedies and orthodox medicine is that orthodox pharmacological drugs are prescribed as a single entity, whereas a herbal prescription will reflect the synergy of the chosen plant remedies and the range of symptoms being presented. In 1978, the German government established the Commission E to investigate and monitor the safety and effectiveness of herbal medicines and a collection of monographs was collated defining their 'reasonable certainty' about the safety and effectiveness of herbs, but while they provide valuable information, they should not be regarded as the definitive source on the subject.

There are several methods of administration within herbal medicine. These include: tablets, infusions (leaves and flowers of a plant are steeped in hot water for 20–30 min and then drained); decoctions (made by boiling the bark, roots or woody sections of a plant, cooling and straining) and tinctures (made by steeping plant material in a preparation of alcohol and water at room temperature for up to 2 weeks). Herbs are classified as 'rising, floating, condensing and sinking', which reflect the cycles of the moon and seasons and according to whether they are 'hot, cold, moist, dry or temperate'. In addition, remedies are classified according to their actions, i.e. warming remedies such as vasodilators and circulatory stimulants; cooling remedies such as relaxants and bitters; diuretics; expectorants; alteratives for detoxification and cleansing; tonic and hormonal remedies; and healing remedies.

Constituents of herbal remedies include:

Alkaloids: the nitrogen-containing constituent, often the basis for orthodox drugs such as morphine and other opiate alkaloids, ergotamine, vincristine and vinblastine.

Flavonoid glycosides: pigments, usually yellow, with specific pharmacological properties, some being diuretic, antispasmodic, antiinflammatory or antiseptic. According to the state of oxygenation, derivatives include: flavones, flavonols and flavonones.

Furanocoumarins: photosensitizing compounds.

Glycosides: secondary plant metabolites which yield one or more sugars on hydrolysis, most commonly glucose.

Isoflavones (phytoestrogens): naturally occurring, weak constituents which bind to oestrogen receptors where they exert an oestrogenic or anti-oestrogenic action depending on the hormonal status of the person.

Mucilages: act as a demulcent, soothing and antiinflammatory agent; may also have incidental healing effects, mainly by trapping water to form a protective gel.

Polysaccharides:   complex units based on sugars and uronic acid, thought to have an important role as immuno-enhancing agents.

Resins:   hard, brittle, secretions which soften on heating, soluble in ether or alcohol, chemically diverse; astringent, may stimulate phagocytic activity.

Saponins:   complex steroidal glycosides, regulate hormonal activity, diuretic, antiinflammatory and digestive effects. Can be toxic if given by injection since they cause haemolysis.

Tannins:   phenolic plant constituents having an astringent effect on the body, obtained from old and dying leaves, traditionally used to tan animal skins.

Volatile oils:   hydrocarbons; may have stimulant, antispasmodic, bitter, carminative, antiseptic and relaxing properties.

Herbal medicines, including essential oils, are also classified according to their therapeutic properties.

Adaptogen:   facilitates adaptability, helping to re-balance and restore homeostasis.

Anti-tussive: suppresses cough reflex.

Astringent:   refers to the binding action of the tannin constituent on mucus membranes to make an antiinfective barrier against external organisms.

Calmative:   induces rest.

Carminative:   reduces flatulence and colic, soothes and settles the gut wall.

Cathartic:   laxative.

Cholagogic:   stimulates flow of bile from the liver.

Circulatory:   stimulates circulation.

Demulcent:   soothing effect on mucous membranes.

Diaphoretic:   stimulates sweat glands by vasodilation.

Digestive tonic:   aids digestion.

Diuretic:   increases diuresis.

Eliminative:   encourages elimination from the body either as a laxative, diuretic, expectorant or diaphoretic.

Emmenagogic:   stimulates uterine bleeding.

Febrifuge:   reduces fever.

Galactogogue:   promotes the secretion of breast milk.

Nervous restoratives:   restores debilitated nervous system following conditions such as depression, nervous exhaustion and general fatigue, some are stimulating and others are relaxing and are used depending on the presenting symptoms.

Vasodilators:   dilates the peripheral blood vessels to improve circulation.

Vulnerary:   aids wound healing.

Safety:   Many people believe that because herbs are natural, they are also safe – and safer than drugs. However, this is not necessarily so and practitioners and patients need to be aware of the potential dangers of mixing herbal remedies with orthodox medication or with other herbs which have similar properties. In addition to their intrinsic therapeutic actions herbal remedies may interfere with the liver's cytochrome P450 enzyme system and its substrates resulting in increased levels of drugs metabolized by this system, for example: the tricyclic antidepressants, antipsychotics, benzodiazepines, oral hypoglycaemic agents, angiotensin 11 receptor antagonists, proton pump inhibitors, warfarin, non-steroidal antiinflammatories including aspirin, antihistamines. Many herbal remedies are known to have anticoagulant effects and patients should discontinue herbal medicine use at least 2 weeks prior to surgery or invasive procedures to avoid interactions with anaesthesia and other drugs and to prevent postoperative haemorrhage. Children, pregnant and lactating women should not use herbal remedies without expert advice. Herbal tinctures contain alcohol, therefore caution is needed if the patient is a recovering alcoholic, taking antabuse or metronidazole.

### Bibliography

Abebe W 2002 Herbal medication: potential for adverse interactions with analgesic drugs. Journal of Clinical Pharmacy and Therapeutics 27(6):391–401

Barnes J, Anderson L, Phillipson J 2002 Herbal Medicines. Pharmaceutical Press, London

Basch E, Ulbricht C 2005 Natural Standard Herb and Supplement Handbook. Mosby, St Louis

Fetrow C, Avila J 2001 Professional's Handbook of Complementary and Alternative Medicines, 2nd edn. Springhouse, Pennsylvania

Gurley B J, Swain A, Hubbard M A et al 2008 Clinical assessment of CYP2D6-mediated herb-drug interactions in humans: effects of milk thistle, black cohosh, goldenseal, kava kava, St. John's wort and Echinacea. Molecular Nutrition and Food Research 52(7):755–763

Healey B, Burgess C, Siebers R 2002 Do natural health food stores require regulation? New Zealand Medical Journal 115(1161):U165

Hellum B H, Nilsen O G 2007 The in vitro inhibitory potential of trade herbal products on human CYP2D6-mediated metabolism and the influence of ethanol. Basic and Clinical Pharmacology and Toxicology 101(5):350–358

Izzo A A, Di Carlo G, Borrelli F et al 2005 Cardiovascular pharmacotherapy and herbal medicines: the risk of drug interaction. International Journal of Cardiology 98(1):1–14

Kleinschmidt S, Rump G, Kotter J 2007 Herbal medications: possible importance for anaesthesia and intensive care medicine. Der Anaesthesist 56(12):1257–1266

Marcus D M, Snodgrass W R 2005 Do no harm: avoidance of herbal medicines during pregnancy. Obstetrics and Gynecology 105(5 Pt 1):1119–1122

Patra K K, Coffey C E 2004 Implications of herbal alternative medicine for electroconvulsive therapy. Journal of ECT 20(3):186–194

Tiran D 2003 The use of herbs by pregnant and childbearing women: a risk-benefit assessment. Complementary Therapies in Nursing and Midwifery 9(4):176–181

Vora C K, Mansoor G A 2005 Herbs and alternative therapies: relevance to hypertension and cardiovascular diseases. Current Hypertension Reports 7(4):275–280

Woodward K N 2005 The potential impact of the use of homeopathic and herbal remedies on monitoring the safety of prescription products. Human Experimental Toxicology 24(5):219–233

Woolf A D 2003 Herbal remedies and children: do they work? Are they harmful? Pediatrics 112(1 Pt 2):240–246

---

Resources

National Institute of Medical Herbalists: www.nihm.org.uk

## Selected herbal remedies

*Agnus castus* (Vitex agnus castus) *(also known as Chasteberry, Chaste tree)*

Traditional uses: as a hormonal remedy for menstrual problems resulting from corpus luteum deficiency, including premenstrual syndrome, dysmenorrhoea and menopausal problems.

Principal constituents: alkaloids, diterpenes, flavonoids, iridoloids.

Evidence: *In vitro*, animal and clinical studies support its effect on follicle stimulating hormone and increasing the release of luteinizing hormone and its effect on premenstrual syndrome, cyclic mastalgia, increased lactation and the treatment of acne.

Safety: Caution regarding concurrent medication, herbs and supplements with similar therapeutic actions, in particular, herbs with diuretic properties which may potentiate the therapeutic effects and concurrent hormonal preparations including the contraceptive pill. Theoretically agnus castus may interfere with dopamine antagonists such as chlorpromazine, haloperidol or fluphenazine.

### Bibliography

Braun L 2006 Chasteberry (Vitex agnus-castus). Journal of Complementary Medicine 5(4):71–73

Daniele C, Thompson Coon J 2005 Vitex agnus castus: a systematic review of adverse events. Drug Safety 28(4):319–332

Dugoua J J, Seely D, Perri D 2008 Safety and efficacy of chaste tree (Vitex agnus-castus) during pregnancy and lactation. Canadian Journal Clinical Pharmacology 15(1):e74–e79

Huddleston M, Jackson E A 2001 Is an extract of the fruit of agnus castus (chaste tree or chasteberry) effective for prevention of symptoms of premenstrual syndrome (PMS)? Journal of Family Practice 50(4):298

Hueneke P 2004 Clinical observations on Vitex and ADHD. Journal of the Australian Traditional Medicine Society 10(1):7–8

Schellenberg R 2001 Treatment for the premenstrual syndrome with agnus castus fruit extract: prospective, randomised, placebo controlled study. British Medical Journal 322(7279):134–137

Webster D E, Lu J, Chen S N 2006 Activation of the mu-opiate receptor by Vitex agnus-castus methanol extracts: implication for its use in PMS. Journal of Ethnopharmacology 106(2):216–221

Wuttke W, Jarry H, Christoffel V 2003 Chaste tree (Vitex agnus-castus) – pharmacology and clinical indications. Phytomedicine 10(4):348–357

*Agrimony* (Agrimonia eupatoria) *(also known as Church steeple, Liverwort, Stickwort)*

Traditional uses: as an astringent, antiseptic, diuretic, used for urinary incontinence, cystitis, gall bladder disease and colic.

Principal constituents: acids, flavonoids, tannins, vitamins.

Evidence: hypoglycaemic, antibacterial (*Staphylococcus aureus*), immunostimulant and gastrointestinal healing properties.

Safety:    May cause lithium toxicity.

Bibliography

Copland A, Nahar L, Tomlinson C T et al 2003 Antibacterial and free radical scavenging activity of the seeds of Agrimonia eupatoria. Fitoterapia 74(1–2): 133–135

Gray A M, Flatt P R 1998 Actions of the traditional anti-diabetic plant, Agrimony eupatoria (agrimony): effects on hyperglycaemia, cellular glucose metabolism and insulin secretion. British Journal of Nutrition 80(1):109–114

Kwon D H, Kwon H Y, Kim H J et al 2005 Inhibition of hepatitis B virus by an aqueous extract of Agrimonia eupatoria L. Phytotherapy Research 19(4):355–358

Li Y, Ooi L S, Wang H et al 2004 Antiviral activities of medicinal herbs traditionally used in southern mainland China. Phytotherapy Research 18(9):718–722

*Aloe vera* (Aloe vera) *(also known as Burn plant, Miracle plant)*

Traditional uses:    as a laxative, healing agent used for wounds, burns, eczema and psoriasis.

Principal constituents:    mono- and polysaccharides, tannins, sterols, organic acids, enzymes, saponins, vitamins and minerals, carbohydrates and lipids.

Evidence:    Has been shown to have wound healing, hypoglycaemic, anticoagulant and antiinflammatory properties.

Safety:    Chronic oral use may result in electrolyte imbalance. Thought to increase the effects of cardiac glycosides and anti-arrhythmic drugs. Internal use contraindicated in renal and cardiac pathology. May increase risk of haemorrhage in patients with bleeding disorders or on anticoagulants, including aspirin and NSAIDs.

Bibliography

Belfrage B, Malmström R 2008 Several cases of liver affected by aloe vera. Lakartidningen 105(1–2):45

Bottenberg M M, Wall G C, Harvey R L et al 2007 Oral aloe vera-induced hepatitis. Annals of Pharmacotherapy 41(10):1740–1743

Choonhakarn C, Busaracome P, Sripanidkulchai B et al 2008 The efficacy of aloe vera gel in the treatment of oral lichen planus: a randomized controlled trial. British Journal of Dermatology 158(3):573–577

Dannemann K, Hecker W, Haberland H 2008 Use of complementary and alternative medicine in children with type 1 diabetes mellitus – prevalence, patterns of use and costs. Pediatric Diabetes 9(3):228–235

Duansak D, Somboonwong J, Patumraj S 2003 Effects of Aloe vera on leukocyte adhesion and TNF-alpha and IL-6 levels in burn wounded rats. Clinical Hemorheology and Microcirculation 29(3-4):239-246

Kirdpon S, Kirdpon W, Airarat W et al 2006 Effect of aloe (Aloe vera Linn.) on healthy adult volunteers: changes in urinary composition. Journal of the Medical Association of Thailand 89(Suppl 2):S9-14

Kim E J, Kim H J, Kim S G 2007 Aloe-induced Henoch-Schonlein purpura. Nephrology (Carlton) 12(1):109

Luyckx V A, Ballantine R, Claeys M et al 2002 Herbal remedy-associated acute renal failure secondary to Cape aloes. American Journal of Kidney Disease 39:E13

Maenthaisong R, Chaiyakunapruk N, Niruntraporn S et al 2007 The efficacy of aloe vera used for burn wound healing: a systematic review. Burns 33(6):713-718

Merchant T E, Bosley C, Smith J 2007 Phase III trial comparing an anionic phospholipid-based cream and aloe vera-based gel in the prevention of radiation dermatitis in pediatric patients. Radiation Oncology 2:45

Reuter J, Jocher A, Stump J 2008 Investigation of the antiinflammatory potential of Aloe vera gel (97.5%) in the ultraviolet erythema test. Skin Pharmacology and Physiology 21(2):106-110

Vogler B K, Ernst E 1999 Aloe vera: a systematic review of its clinical effectiveness. British Journal of General Practice 49:823-828

## Angelica (Angelica sinensis) *(also known as Dong quai)*

**Traditional uses:** as a digestive tonic, antispasmodic, expectorant, diuretic, local antiinflammatory properties used for debilitating illnesses, hepatic conditions, asthma, paediatric respiratory conditions.

**Principal constituents:** coumarins, tannins, resin.

**Evidence:** Studies indicate that angelica is antiinflammatory, anticoagulant, antimicrobial (*Escherichia coli, Streptococcus faecalis, Salmonella typhi*).

**Safety:** May increase the risk of bleeding in patients with bleeding disorders and potentiate the effects of anticoagulants, including aspirin and NSAIDs. May increase the effects of beta blockers, calcium channel blockers and digoxin.

---

### Bibliography

Anonymous 2004 Angelica sinensis (Dong quai). Alternative Medical Review 9(4):429-433

Astegiano M, Pellicano R, Terzi E 2006 Treatment of irritable bowel syndrome: a case control experience. Minerva Gastroenterologica e Dietologica 52(4): 359-363

Cheema D, Coomarasamy A, El-Toukhy T 2007 Non-hormonal therapy of post-menopausal vasomotor symptoms: a structured evidence-based review. Archives of Gynecology and Obstetrics Review 276(5):463–469

Gu Q, Xu J Y, Cheng L G et al 2007 The effect of Angelica sinensis on adhesion, invasion, migration and metastasis of melanoma cells. Zhong Yao Cai 30(3): 302–305

Lu J, Kim S H, Jiang C et al 2007 Oriental herbs as a source of novel anti-androgen and prostate cancer chemopreventive agents. Acta Pharmacology Sinese 28(9): 1365–1372

Piersen C E 2003 Phytoestrogens in botanical dietary supplements: implications for cancer. Integrative Cancer Therapies 2(2):120–138

Xin Y F, Zhou G L, Shen M et al 2007 Angelica sinensis: a novel adjunct to prevent doxorubicin-induced chronic cardiotoxicity. Basic Clinical Pharmacology Toxicology 101(6):421–426

## *Arnica* (Arnica montana) *(also known as Leopards bane, Wolf's bane)*

Traditional uses:    local healing, stimulates peripheral blood supply.

Principal constituents:    alkaloids, amines, coumarins, terpenoids, flavonoids.

Evidence:    Has been shown to be antiinflammatory, antimicrobial (*Listeria monocytogenes Salmonella typhimurium, Staphylococcus aureus, Proteus vulgaris, Trichophyton mentagrophytes*).

Safety:    For topical application only, not for oral use. It is necessary also to differentiate between the herbal (i.e. pharmacological) preparation and the homeopathic (i.e. highly diluted) remedy.

### Bibliography

Kouzi S A, Nuzum D S 2007 Arnica for bruising and swelling. American Journal of Health-System Pharmacy 64(23):2434–2443

Lass C, Vocanson M, Wagner S et al 2008 Anti-inflammatory and immune-regulatory mechanisms prevent contact hypersensitivity to Arnica montana L. Experimental Dermatology 12 March, [Epub ahead of print]

Widrig R, Suter A, Saller R et al 2007 Choosing between NSAID and arnica for topical treatment of hand osteoarthritis in a randomised, double-blind study. Rheumatology International 27(6):585–591

## *Astragalus* (Astragalus branaceous) *(also known as Huang chi, Milk vetch)*

Traditional uses:    Used in traditional Chinese medicine to enhance the immune system, diuretic.

Principal constituents: betaine, betasitoserol choline, glycosides, saponins, polysaccharides.

Evidence: Trials indicate that astragalus may be antiinflammatory, hypotensive, diuretic, hypoglycaemic, antiviral, antioxidant and have muscle-repairing properties.

Safety: May interfere with immunosuppressive therapy, contraindicated in transplant surgery. May increase the risk of bleeding in patients with bleeding disorders and potentiate the effects of anticoagulants. Contraindicated in diabetics. May increase the effects of paralytics such as pancuronium and succinylcholine.

Bibliography

Ahmed M S, Hou S H, Battaglia M C 2007 Treatment of idiopathic membranous nephropathy with the herb Astragalus membranaceus. American Journal of Kidney Disease 50(6):1028–1032

Ho J W, Jie M 2007 Pharmacological activity of cardiovascular agents from herbal medicine. Cardiovascular Hematology Agents in Medical Chemistry 5(4):273–277

Lee H-J, Lee J-H 2005 Effects of medicinal herb tea on the smoking cessation and reducing smoking withdrawal symptoms. American Journal of Chinese Medicine 33(1):127–138

Wang G, Liu C T, Wang Z L 2005 Effects of Astragalus membranaceus in promoting T-helper cell type 1 polarization and interferon-gamma production by up-regulating T-bet expression in patients with asthma. Chinese Journal of Integrative Medicine 12(4):262–267

*Bearberry* (Uva ursi)

Traditional uses: urinary tract antiseptic, diuretic, used for urinary tract infections.

Principal constituents: flavonoids, quinines, tannins, terpenoids.

Evidence: Bearberry has been shown to be antiseptic, antimicrobial (*Escherichia coli*), antioxidant and diuretic.

Safety: As bearberry is known to inhibit melanin synthesis, caution should be used; one case report indicates possible toxicity affecting the retina.

Bibliography

Bousová I, Martin J, Jahodár L et al 2005 Evaluation of in vitro effects of natural substances of plant origin using a model of protein glycoxidation. Journal of Pharmaceutical and Biomedical Analysis 37(5):957–962

Cervenka L, Peskova I, Foltynova E et al 2006 Inhibitory effects of some spice and herb extracts against Arcobacter butzleri, A. cryaerophilus and A. skirrowii. Current Microbiology 53(5):435–439

Chauhan B, Yu C, Krantis A et al 2007 In vitro activity of uva-ursi against cytochrome P450 isoenzymes and P-glycoprotein. Canadian Journal Physiology Pharmacology 85(11):1099–1107

Wang L, Del Priore L V 2004 Bull's-eye maculopathy secondary to herbal toxicity from uva ursi. American Journal of Ophthalmology 137(6):1135–1137

Yarnell E 2002 Botanical medicines for the urinary tract. World Journal of Urology 20(5):285–293

Newton M, Combest W, Kosier J H 2001 Select herbal remedies used to treat common urologic conditions. Urology Nursing 21(3):232–234

## Bilberry (Vaccinium myrtillus) (also known as Huckleberry, Whortleberry, Wineberry)

Traditional uses:   for ophthalmic conditions such as to improve visual acuity, for cataracts and retinal conditions; for circulatory problems including varicose veins, atherosclerosis, venous insufficiency and haemorrhoids. It is also used orally for gastrointestinal and urinary disorders. Topically, it is used for inflammation of the mucous membranes in the mouth and throat.

Principal constituents:   anthocyanosides, tannins, flavonoids.

Evidence:   Some studies indicate that bilberry is cholesterol reducing, hypoglycaemic, antispasmodic, antibacterial (*Staphylococcus aureus*, *Escherichia coli*, *Helicobacter pylori*) and affects platelet aggregation. There is some thought that it may improve diabetic retinopathy.

Safety:   Bilberry may increase the risk of bleeding in patients with bleeding disorders and potentiate the effects of anticoagulants, aspirin and non-steroidal antiinflammatory drugs. Avoid in pregnancy as there is insufficient information available on the teratogenic effects. As bilberry may have the potential to lower blood glucose, caution is needed in diabetic patients taking medication to control blood glucose levels.

### Bibliography

Chatterjee A, Yasmin T, Bagchi D et al 2004 Inhibition of Helicobacter pylori in vitro by various berry extracts, with enhanced susceptibility to clarithromycin. Molecular Cell Biochemistry 265(1–2):19–26

Choi E H, Ok H E, Yoon Y 2007 Protective effect of anthocyanin-rich extract from bilberry (Vaccinium myrtillus L.) against myelotoxicity induced by 5-fluorouracil. Biofactors 29(1):55–65

Kiser A K, Dagnelie G 2008 Reported effects of non-traditional treatments and complementary and alternative medicine by retinitis pigmentosa patients. Clinical Experimental Optometry 91(2):166–176

Muth E-R, Laurent J-M, Jasper P 2000 The effect of bilberry nutritional supplementation on night visual acuity and contrast sensitivity. Alternative Medical Review 5(2):164–173

Zafra-Stone S, Yasmin T, Bagchi M 2007 Berry anthocyanins as novel antioxidants in human health and disease prevention. Molecular Nutrition Food Research Review 51(6):675–683

*Black cohosh* (Cimicifuga racemosa) *(also known as Black snakeroot, Baneberry, Bugwort, Cimicifuga, Phytoestrogen, Rattleweed, Sheng ma, squaw root)*

Traditional uses:   Popular contemporary use of black cohosh is as a natural form of hormone replacement therapy in the perimenopausal period and for dysmenorrhoea, but it has also been used as an antispasmodic, antiinflammatory and as a vasodilator for muscle cramps and tension.

Principal constituents:  alkaloids, tannins, terpenoids, cimicifugin, racemosin, salicylic acid.

Evidence:   *In vitro* animal studies and clinical trials indicates hormonal, antiinflammatory, anticoagulant, hypotensive, analgesic and antibacterial (v. *Staphylococcus aureus, Escherichia coli*) properties.

Safety:   Avoid in pregnancy until term, as it may trigger uterine contractions. Black cohosh may increase risk of bleeding in patients with bleeding disorders or in those on anticoagulants including aspirin and non-steroidal antiinflammatories. May increase the effects of oestrogen supplements and should be avoided in those with hormone-sensitive conditions. There is some evidence to suggest that it may increase metastatic growth in women with breast cancer; caution should be used in women taking Tamoxifen. May be hepatotoxic in large doses or if taken concurrently with medication which has hepatotoxic side-effects. Care should be taken not to confuse black cohosh with blue cohosh (*Caulophyllum thalictroides*).

Bibliography

Baillie N, Rasmussen P 1997 Black and blue cohosh in labour. New Zealand Medical Journal 110:20–21

Chitturi S, Farrell G C 2008 Hepatotoxic slimming aids and other herbal hepatotoxins. Journal of Gastroenterology Hepatology 23(3):366–373

Cohen S et al 2004 Immune hepatitis associated with use of black cohosh: case study. Menopause 11:575–577

Davis V L, Jayo M J, Hardy M L et al 2003 Effects of black cohosh on mammary tumor development and progression in MMTV-neu transgenic mice. 94th Annual Meeting of the American Association for Cancer Research, Washington DC

Farnsworth N R, Krause E C, Bolton J L 2008 The University of Illinois at Chicago/National Institutes of Health Center for Botanical Dietary Supplements Research for Women's Health: from plant to clinical use. American Journal of Clinical Nutrition 87(2):504S–508S

Gurley B J, Swain A, Hubbard M A et al 2008 Clinical assessment of CYP2D6-mediated herb-drug interactions in humans: effects of milk thistle, black cohosh, goldenseal, kava kava, St. John's wort and Echinacea. Molecular Nutrition and Food Research 52(7):755–763

Joy D, Joy J, Duane P 2008 Black cohosh: a cause of abnormal postmenopausal liver function tests. Climacteric 11(1):84–88

Mahady G B, Low Dog T, Barrett M L et al 2008 United States Pharmacopeia review of the black cohosh case reports of hepatotoxicity. Menopause 15(4 Part 1): 628–638

Nisbet B C, O'Connor R E 2007 Black cohosh-induced hepatitis. Delaware Medical Journal 79(11):441–444

Ruhlen R L, Haubner J, Tracy J K et al 2007 Black cohosh does not exert an estrogenic effect on the breast. Nutrition Cancer 59(2):269–277

Vitetta L, Thomsen M, Sali A 2003 Black cohosh and other herbal remedies associated with acute hepatitis. Medical Journal of Australia 178:411–412

*Blue cohosh* (Caulophyllum thalictroides) *(also known as Blue ginseng, Caulophyllum, Papoose root, Squaw root)*

Traditional uses:   The primary use of blue cohosh is to stimulate the uterus to induce labour or menstruation, but it is also used as an antispasmodic, laxative and for rheumatic conditions.

Principal constituents:   steroidal saponins, alkaloids, magnoflorine, cystine, laburnine, taspine.

Evidence:   There is considerable evidence of the uterine-stimulating properties of blue cohosh and of its potential side-effects.

Safety: Blue cohosh is a uterine stimulant and several constituents are potentially teratogenic; use of blue cohosh in pregnancy, especially towards term, can cause life-threatening toxicity in the infant, including stroke and death. Although many nurse-midwives in the USA and some mothers in both the USA and in the UK use blue cohosh to facilitate the onset of labour, they should be advised that this is dangerous; the National Institute of Medical Herbalists in the UK strongly discourages the use of blue cohosh. The taspine constituent is chemically similar to morphine – should not be taken concurrently with morphine and morphine-derivative medications. It may also decrease the effectiveness of anti-diabetic and anti-hypertensive medications. It should be avoided in anyone with a cardiac condition.

Bibliography

Dugoua J J, Perri D, Seely D 2008 Safety and efficacy of blue cohosh (Caulophyllum thalictroides) during pregnancy and lactation. Canadian Journal of Clinical Pharmacology 15(1):e66–e73
Edmunds J 1999 Blue cohosh and newborn myocardial infarction? Midwifery Today with International Midwife(52):34–35
Finkel R S, Zarlengo K M 2004 Blue cohosh and perinatal stroke. New England Journal of Medicine 351(3):302–303
Jones T K, Lawson B M 1998 Profound neonatal congestive heart failure caused by maternal consumption of blue cohosh herbal medication. Journal of Pediatrics 132(3 Pt 1):550–552

## Boldo (Peumus boldus)

Traditional uses: as a digestive and hepatobiliary remedy and for colds, gout, headache, menstrual pain.

Principal constituents: alkaloids, flavonoids, volatile oil, coumarin, resin and tannin.

Evidence: Studies indicate diuretic, muscle relaxant, anticoagulant, antioxidant and central nervous system (CNS) inhibition.

Safety: Boldo is contraindicated in CNS or respiratory disorders and should not be taken concurrently with sedation or with analgesics containing codeine. It may increase the risk of bleeding in patients with bleeding disorders or taking anticoagulants including aspirin and NSAIDs. Boldo has been shown to be hepatotoxic.

Bibliography

Izzo A A, Di Carlo G, Borrelli F et al 2005 Cardiovascular pharmacotherapy and herbal medicines: the risk of drug interaction. International Journal of Cardiology 98(1):1–14

Lambert J P, Cormier J 2001 Potential interaction between warfarin and boldo-fenugreek. Pharmacotherapy 21(4):509–512

Monzón S, Lezaun A, Sáenz D et al 2004 Anaphylaxis to boldo infusion, a herbal remedy. Allergy 59(9):1019–1020

O'Brien P, Carrasco-Pozo C, Speisky H 2006 Boldine and its antioxidant or health-promoting properties. Chemico-biological Interactions 159(1):1–17

Piscaglia F, Leoni S, Venturi A et al 2005 Caution in the use of boldo in herbal laxatives: a case of hepatotoxicity. Scandinavian Journal of Gastroenterology 40(2):236–239

## Boneset (Eupatorium perfoliatum) *(also known as Fever wort, Agueweed)*

Traditional uses:    Boneset has been used for influenza, acute bronchitis, nasopharyngeal conditions, as a urinary tract antiseptic and diuretic.

Principal constituents:    flavonoids, volatile oil, terpenoids.

Evidence:    Non-clinical studies indicate that boneset may have antibacterial, immunostimulant and antiinflammatory properties.

Safety:    Allergic reactions have been reported, notably in people allergic to chrysanthemums, marigolds and daisies. It is important to avoid confusion with gravel root (*Eupatorium purpureum*), also known as boneset.

Bibliography

Habtemariam S, Macpherson A M 2000 Cytotoxicity and antibacterial activity of ethanol extract from leaves of a herbal drug, boneset (Eupatorium perfoliatum). Phytotherapy Research 4:575–577

## Borage (Borago officinalis) *(also known as Starflower oil)*

Traditional uses:    Borage seed oil is used for rheumatoid arthritis, atopic eczema, seborrhoeic dermatitis in babies and stress. It is particularly popular for premenstrual syndrome and has been used for attention deficit-hyperactivity disorder (ADHD), alcoholism, depression, reducing pyrexia and for preventing heart disease and stroke. Borage is also used as a cardiac tonic, sedative and to increase circulatory capacity and breast milk production.

Principal constituents: Borage oil contains 18–26% gamma-linolenic acid, an omega-6 fatty acid but the leaves and flowers do not. Alkaloids and mucilages are the other main constituents.

Evidence: Studies indicate that borage oil has antiinflammatory, central nervous system stimulating and anticoagulant effects.

Safety: Certain constituents in borage are potentially pneumotoxic, carcinogenic, hepatotoxic and mutagenic. It may decrease efficacy of anticonvulsive therapy, increases risk of temporal lobe epilepsy in schizophrenics. It may also increase bleeding in people with bleeding disorders or in those taking anticoagulants.

Bibliography

Conforti F, Sosa S, Marrelli M 2008 In vivo antiinflammatory and in vitro antioxidant activities of Mediterranean dietary plants. Journal of Ethnopharmacology 116(1):144–151

Gilani A H, Bashir S, Khan A U 2007 Pharmacological basis for the use of Borago officinalis in gastrointestinal, respiratory and cardiovascular disorders. Journal of Ethnopharmacology 114(3):393–399

Kanehara S, Ohtani T, Uede K et al 2007 Clinical effects of undershirts coated with borage oil on children with atopic dermatitis: a double-blind, placebo-controlled clinical trial. Journal of Dermatology 34(12):811–815

*Broom* (Sarothamnus scoparius) *(also known as Sorghum)*

Traditional uses: Primarily used for digestive disorders, but also as a peripheral vasoconstrictor and for oedema associated with heart failure.

Principal constituents: alkaloids, sparteine, genistein, flavonoids, volatile oil, thiamine, riboflavin, cyanogenic glycosides.

Evidence: Animal studies indicate cardiotoxic properties.

Safety: Increases the effect of beta-blockers and may cause serious arrhythmias; may interfere with cardiac pacemakers and may decrease the effectiveness of anti-hypertensive therapy.

Bibliography

Nirmal J, Babu C S, Harisudhan T et al 2008 Evaluation of behavioural and antioxidant activity of Cytisus scoparius Link in rats exposed to chronic unpredictable mild stress. BMC Complementary and Alternative Medicine 8:15

Raja S, Ahamed K F, Kumar V et al 2007 Antioxidant effect of Cytisus scoparius against carbon tetrachloride treated liver injury in rats. Journal of Ethnopharmacology 109(1):41–47

Sundararajan R, Haja N A, Venkatesan K et al 2006 Cytisus scoparius link – a natural antioxidant. BMC Complementary and Alternative Medicine 6:8

## Buchu (Barosma betulina)

Traditional uses:   as an antiinflammatory, antiseptic and diuretic, for urinary tract infections and for sexually transmitted diseases.

Principal constituents:   volatile oil, glycosides, flavonoids, resin, mucilage, diosphenol.

Evidence:   Non-clinical studies indicate antiinflammatory, abortifacient and anticoagulant properties.

Safety:   Avoid concomitant use with drugs and other herbs with diuretic properties, which may potentiate the effect. Buchu is thought to increase the effect of cardiac glycosides. It may increase the risk of bleeding in patients with bleeding disorders or taking anticoagulants and is thought to be abortifacient. Can cause gastrointestinal and renal irritation.

### Bibliography

Simpson D 1998 Buchu – South Africa's amazing herbal remedy. Scottish Medical Journal 43(6):189–191

## Burdock (Arctium lappa)

Traditional uses:   as a diuretic, laxative, antiinflammatory, for skin conditions such as eczema and as an antibiotic.

Principal constituents:   inulin, glycosides, flavonoids, tannin, volatile oil, mucilage, pectin and sugars.

Evidence:   In vitro research indicates antimicrobial (Staphylococcus aureus, Escherichia coli), anticoagulant, uterine stimulant, diuretic, hyper/hypoglycaemic and antipyretic properties.

Safety:   Avoid concomitant use with drugs and other herbs with diuretic properties which may potentiate the effects. Burdock has been known to be contaminated by atropine in commercial form. Burdock may increase the risk of bleeding in patients with bleeding disorders or taking anticoagulants. Caution in hormone sensitive conditions including HRT. May cause allergic reactions in those allergic to chrysanthemums, marigolds and daisies.

Bibliography

Holetz F B, Pessini G L, Sanches N R et al 2002 Screening of some plants used in the Brazilian folk medicine for the treatment of infectious diseases. Memórias do Instituto Oswaldo Cruz 97:1027–1031

Cicero A F, Derosa G, Gaddi A 2004 What do herbalists suggest to diabetic patients in order to improve glycemic control? Evaluation of scientific evidence and potential risks. Acta Diabetologia 41(3):91–98

## Butcher's broom (Ruscus aculeatus) *(also known as Sweet broom)*

Traditional uses:  Butcher's broom has been used for haemorrhoids, gallstones, atherosclerosis, symptoms of chronic venous insufficiency, as a laxative, diuretic, antiinflammatory and to facilitate wound healing in fractures.

Principal constituents:  steroidal saponins, ruscogenin and neoruscogenin, coumarins, flavonoids and tryamine.

Evidence:  Some studies indicate antiinflammatory and vasoconstrictive (hypertensive) properties while others demonstrate a possible anti-hypertensive effect.

Safety:  Butcher's broom should not be taken concomitantly with diuretics, anti-hypertensive medication or anticoagulants. As it contains tyramine, it should be avoided in those taking monoamine oxidase inhibitors. Take care not to confuse butcher's broom with Scotch broom or Spanish broom.

Bibliography

Beltramino R, Penenory A, Buceta A M 2000 An open-label, randomized multicenter study comparing the efficacy and safety of Cyclo 3 Fort versus hydroxyethyl rutoside in chronic venous lymphatic insufficiency. Angiology 51:535–544

Redman D A 2000 Ruscus aculeatus (butcher's broom) as a potential treatment for orthostatic hypotension, with a case report. Journal of Alternative and Complementary Medicine 6:539–549

Vanscheidt W, Jost V, Wolna P et al 2002 Efficacy and safety of a Butcher's broom preparation (Ruscus aculeatus L. extract) compared to placebo in patients suffering from chronic venous insufficiency. Arzneimittelforschung 52:243–250

*Calamus* (Acorus calamus) *(also known as Sweet flag, Flagroot, Kalmus, Sweet grass)*

Traditional uses:    Calamus has been used for dyspepsia, hyperacidity, colic, flatulence, peptic ulceration and for anorexia.

Principal constituents:    volatile oil, amines, bitter, resin, tannin and mucilages.

Evidence:    Studies indicate antiinflammatory and vasoconstrictive (hypertensive) properties and more recently, antibacterial effects.

Safety:    Caution regarding concurrent sedation and analgesics containing codeine. May increase stomach acid and reduce the effectiveness of antacids. Contraindicated in psychiatric illness. May potentiate monoamine oxidase inhibitors.

Bibliography

Acuña U M, Atha D E, Ma J et al 2002 Antioxidant capacities of ten edible North American plants. Phytotherapy Research 16(1):63–65

Ahmad I, Aqil F 2007 In vitro efficacy of bioactive extracts of 15 medicinal plants against ESbetaL-producing multidrug-resistant enteric bacteria. Microbiological Research 162(3):264–275

Aqil F, Ahmad I 2007 Antibacterial properties of traditionally used Indian medicinal plants. Methods and Findings in Experimental and Clinical Pharmacology 29(2):79–92

Aqil F, Ahmad I, Owais M 2006 Evaluation of anti-methicillin-resistant Staphylococcus aureus (MRSA) activity and synergy of some bioactive plant extracts. Biotechnology Journal 1(10):1093–1102

Gilani A U, Shah A J, Ahmad M et al 2006 Antispasmodic effect of Acorus calamus Linn is mediated through calcium channel blockade. Phytotherapy Research 20(12):1080–1084

Mukherjee P K, Kumar V, Mal M et al 2007 In vitro acetylcholinesterase inhibitory activity of the essential oil from Acorus calamus and its main constituents. Planta Medica 73(3):283–285

*Calendula* (Calendula officinalis, Marigold)

Traditional uses:    as a digestive, antiinflammatory, antimicrobial and antispasmodic, used topically for skin conditions and wound healing.

Principal constituents:    flavonoids, polysaccharides, terpenoids, volatile oils.

Evidence:    Calendula has been shown to be antiinflammatory, antimicrobial and antiviral and clinical trials support is use in wound healing.

Safety: Calendula is contraindicated in transplant surgery due to immunostimulant effect. It is a CNS depressant and may cause hypoglycaemia and hypotension if taken orally.

### Bibliography

Basch E, Bent S, Foppa I et al 2006 Marigold (Calendula officinalis L.): an evidence-based systematic review by the Natural Standard Research Collaboration. Journal of Herbal Pharmacotherapy 6(3–4):135–159

Gorchakova T V, Suprun I V, Sobenin I A et al 2007 Use of natural products in anticytokine therapy. Bulletin Experimental Biological Medicine 143(3):316–319

Guala A, Oberle D, Ramos M 2007 Efficacy and safety of two baby creams in children with diaper dermatitis: results of a postmarketing surveillance study. Journal of Alternative and Complementary Medicine 13(1):16–18

McQuestion M 2006 Evidence-based skin care management in radiation therapy. Seminars in Oncology Nursing 22(3):163–173

Ukiya M, Akihisa T, Yasukawa K 2006 Antiinflammatory, anti-tumor-promoting and cytotoxic activities of constituents of marigold (Calendula officinalis) flowers. Journal of Natural Products 69(12):1692–1696

## Cat's claw (Uncaria tomentosa)

Traditional uses: as an antiinflammatory, antiviral, immunostimulant, used for rheumatism, gonorrhoea, gastric ulcers and tumours.

Principal constituents: alkaloids, glycosides.

Evidence: Studies indicate antiinflammatory, anti-tumour, hypotensive, anticoagulant and immunostimulating properties. It may also have a part to play in the treatment of rheumatoid arthritis.

Safety: Contraindicated in transplant surgery due to immunostimulant effects; may increase bleeding in patients with bleeding disorders or on anticoagulants. Should not be confused with Cat's foot.

### Bibliography

Mur E, Hartig F, Eibl G et al 2002 Randomized double blind trial of an extract from the pentacyclic alkaloid-chemotype of Uncaria tomentosa for the treatment of rheumatoid arthritis. Journal of Rheumatology 29:678–681

Piscoya J, Rodriguez Z, Bustamante S A et al 2001 Efficacy and safety of freeze-dried cat's claw in osteoarthritis of the knee: mechanisms of action of the species Uncaria guianensis. Inflammatory Research 50:442–448

Sandoval M, Charbonnet R M, Okuhama N N et al 2000 Cat's claw inhibits TNFalpha production and scavenges free radicals: role in cytoprotection. Free Radical Biology and Medicine 29:71–78

Styczynski J, Wysocki M 2006 Alternative medicine remedies might stimulate viability of leukemic cells. Pediatric Blood Cancer 46:94–98

## Celery (Apium graveolens)

Traditional uses:   Celery has a long history of treatment for gout, headache, weight loss and poor appetite. It is also used as a sedative, mild diuretic, urinary antiseptic, digestive aid, menstrual stimulant, to reduce lactation and for purifying the blood.

Principal constituents: volatile oil, bergapten, flavonoids, furano-coumarins, high in minerals including sodium.

Evidence:   *In vitro* research indicates antispasmodic, sedative and bacteriostatic (v. *Staphylococcus aureus, Vibrio cholerae, Shigella dysenteriae, Streptococcus faecalis, Streptococcus pyrogenes*), hypoglycaemic, hypotensive CNS depressant and anticoagulant properties.

Safety:   Celery can cause allergic and anaphylactic reactions and contact dermatitis. It may inhibit thyroxin medication.

### Bibliography

Chu Y F, Sun J, Wu X et al 2002 Antioxidant and antiproliferative activities of common vegetables. Journal of Agricultural and Food Chemistry 50(23):6910–6916

Heck A M, DeWitt B A, Lukes A L 2000 Potential interactions between alternative therapies and warfarin. American Journal of Health-System Pharmacy 57(13): 1221–1227

Jacovljevic V, Raskovic A, Popovic M et al 2002 The effect of celery and parsley juices on pharmacodynamic activity of drugs involving cytochrome P450 in their metabolism. European Journal of Drug Metabolism Pharmacokinetics 27(3):153–156

Moses G 2001 Thyroxine interacts with celery seed tablets? Australian Prescriber 24:6–7

## Centaury (Centaurium erythraea)

Traditional uses:   as a digestive aid, used for anorexia.

Principal constituents: alkaloids, polyphenolic compounds, monoterpenoids, bitter glycosides, volatile oil, resin, flavonoids.

Evidence:   Studies indicate antiinflammatory, CNS depressant and antipyretic activity and, more recently, antioxidant effects.

Safety: Caution regarding concurrent medication, herbs and supplements with similar therapeutic action, in particular, herbs with diuretic properties which may potentiate effect. Caution regarding concurrent sedation, including analgesics containing codeine. Contraindicated for patients with peptic ulcers.

Bibliography

Valentão P, Fernandes E, Carvalho F et al 2003 Hydroxyl radical and hypochlorous acid scavenging activity of small centaury (Centaurium erythraea) infusion: a comparative study with green tea (Camellia sinensis). Phytomedicine 10(6–7):517–522

## Chamomile (German) (Matricaria recutita)

Traditional uses: Chamomile has a long history as a sedative, an antispasmodic for menstrual cramps, labour pain and intestinal colic. It is also used as an antiinflammatory and antiseptic, particularly for wound healing and for a range of digestive complaints. In inhalation it is useful for respiratory conditions and topically for mucous membrane irritation.

Principal constituents: coumarins, flavonoids, volatile oil.

Evidence: In vitro and animal studies indicate antiinflammatory, anti-allergic, CNS depressant and anticoagulant properties. Clinical trials support its use in wound healing and as a sedative and antispasmodic.

Safety: German chamomile may increase bleeding in patients with bleeding disorders or taking anticoagulants; it may interfere with the liver's cytochrome P450 enzyme system and its substrates resulting in increased levels of drugs metabolized by this system for example: the tricyclic antidepressants, antipsychotics, benzodiazepines, proton pump inhibitors, oral hypoglycaemic agents, angiotensin 11 receptor antagonists and antihistamines. It may have some mild oestrogenic activity, therefore caution with hormone replacement therapy and avoid concomitant use with tamoxifen. German chamomile should not be confused with Roman chamomile which has different constituents.

Bibliography

Bianco M I, Lúquez C, de Jong L I et al 2008 Presence of Clostridium botulinum spores in Matricaria chamomilla (chamomile) and its relationship with infant botulism. International Journal of Food Microbiology 121(3):357–360
Block K I, Gyllenhaal C, Mead M N 2004 Safety and efficacy of herbal sedatives in cancer care. Integrative Cancer Therapies 3(2):128–148

Cuzzolin L, Francini-Pesenti F, Zaffani S et al 2007 Knowledges about herbal products among subjects on warfarin therapy and patient-physician relationship: a pilot study. Pharmacoepidemiology Drug Safety 16(9):1014–1017

Kassi E, Papoutsi Z, Fokialakis N et al 2004 Greek plant extracts exhibit selective estrogen receptor modulator (SERM)-like properties. Journal of Agricultural and Food Chemistry 52:6956–6961

Madisch A, Holtmann G, Mayr G et al 2004 Treatment of functional dyspepsia with a herbal preparation: a double-blind, randomized, placebo-controlled, multicenter trial. Digestion 69:45–52

Maliakal P P, Wanwimolruk S 2001 Effect of herbal teas on hepatic drug metabolizing enzymes in rats. Journal of Pharmacy and Pharmacology 53:1323–1329

Segal R, Pilote L 2006 Warfarin interaction with Matricaria chamomilla. Canadian Medical Association Journal 174:1281–1282

Talhouk R S, Karam C, Fostok S et al 2007 Antiinflammatory bioactivities in plant extracts. Journal Medicinal Food 10(1):1–10

## Coltsfoot (Tussilago farfara) *(also known as Coughwort, Horsehoof)*

Traditional uses:   Traditionally, people have used coltsfoot as a relaxant, expectorant, anti-tussive, demulcent and antimicrobial. It can be applied locally as a healing and soothing remedy for skin problems and wounds. Coltsfoot has also been used to treat asthma and dry coughs.

Principal constituents:   alkaloids, mucilage, tannins, hormonal substances, flavonoids, carotenoids.

Evidence:   Studies have shown coltsfoot to be antiinfective (*Staphylococcus aureus, Bordetella pertussis, Pseudomonas aeruginosa, Proteus vulgaris*), anticoagulant and hypertensive and antioxidant.

Safety:   Contraindicated in hypertensive patients receiving medication, hepatic disease, cardiovascular pathology and those on anticoagulants or with a haemorrhagic disorder. There is some suggestion that coltsfoot may be potentially carcinogenic.

### Bibliography

Cho J, Kim H M, Ryu J H et al 2005 Neuroprotective and antioxidant effects of the ethyl acetate fraction prepared from Tussilago farfara L. Biological and Pharmaceutical Bulletin 28(3):455–460

Chou M W, Fu P P 2006 Formation of DHP-derived DNA adducts in vivo from dietary supplements and Chinese herbal plant extracts containing carcinogenic pyrrolizidine alkaloids. Toxicology and Industrial Health 22(8):321–327

Kim M R, Lee J Y, Lee H H et al 2006 Antioxidative effects of quercetin-glycosides isolated from the flower buds of Tussilago farfara L. Food and Chemical Toxicology 44(8):1299–1307

## Comfrey (Symphytum officinale) *(also known as Knitbone, Boneset)*

Traditional uses:   Comfrey is well known as a remedy for wound healing, but is also used for gastritis, colitis, gastric and duodenal ulcers and as an astringent.

Principal constituents:   alkaloids, gum, mucilage, tannins, triterpenes and allantoin.

Evidence:   Clinical and non-clinical studies indicate a favourable effect on wound healing, when compared to pharmacological preparations, also antiinflammatory and analgesic properties.

Safety:   Comfrey may be hepatotoxic; it is not recommended for oral use.

### Bibliography

D'Anchise R, Bulitta M, Giannetti B 2007 Comfrey extract ointment in comparison to diclofenac gel in the treatment of acute unilateral ankle sprains (distortions). Arzneimittelforschung 57(11):712–716

Dasgupta A 2003 Review of abnormal laboratory test results and toxic effects due to use of herbal medicines. American Journal of Clinical Pathology 120(1):127–137

Grube B, Grünwald J, Krug L et al 2007 Efficacy of a comfrey root (Symphyti offic. radix) extract ointment in the treatment of patients with painful osteoarthritis of the knee: results of a double-blind, randomised, bicenter, placebo-controlled trial. Phytomedicine 14(1):2–10

Koll R, Buhr M, Dieter R et al 2004 Efficacy and tolerance of a comfrey root extract (Extr. Rad. Symphyti) in the treatment of ankle distorsions: results of a multicenter, randomized, placebo-controlled, double-blind study. Phytomedicine 11(6):470–477

Kucera M, Barna M, Horàcek O et al 2005 Topical symphytum herb concentrate cream against myalgia: a randomized controlled double-blind clinical study. Advances in Therapy 22(6):681–692

Stickel F, Seitz H K 2000 The efficacy and safety of comfrey. Public Health Nutrition(4A):501–508

Mei N, Guo L, Zhang L et al 2006 Analysis of gene expression changes in relation to toxicity and tumorigenesis in the livers of Big Blue transgenic rats fed comfrey (Symphytum officinale). BMC Bioinformatics 7(Suppl 2):S16

## Corn silk (Zea mays)

Traditional uses:   Used as a diuretic, for cystitis, prostatitis and urethritis.

Principal constituents: amines, saponins, tannins, resin.

Evidence: Animal studies and some clinical trials indicate hypotensive, hypoglycaemic, anticoagulant and diuretic properties.

Safety: Caution regarding concurrent medication, herbs and supplements with similar therapeutic action, in particular other herbs with diuretic properties, which may potentiate the diuretic effects. Contraindicated in patients with clotting disorders or on anticoagulants.

### Bibliography

Maksimovic Z, Dobric S, Kovacevic N et al 2004 Diuretic activity of Maydis stigma extract in rats. Pharmazie 59(12):967–971

Martins H M, Martins M L, Dias M I et al 2001 Evaluation of microbiological quality of medicinal plants used in natural infusions. International Journal of Food Microbiology 68(1–2):149–153

Rau O, Wurglics M, Dingermann T et al 2006 Screening of herbal extracts for activation of the human peroxisome proliferator-activated receptor. Pharmazie 61(11):952–956

*Couch grass* (Agropyron repens) *(also known as Wheat grass, Dog grass)*

Traditional uses: Used mostly for its concentrated nutrients, to treat conditions such as anaemia, diabetes and enhancing the immune system to facilitate wound healing, but is also used as a diuretic for urinary tract infections, prostatic hypertrophy and urinary tract inflammation. It has also been used as an alternative cancer treatment due to its high chlorophyll content.

Principal constituents: chlorophyll, vitamin A, vitamin C, vitamin E, iron, calcium, magnesium, amino acids, cyanogenetic glycosides, flavonoids, saponins, volatile oils.

Evidence: It is possible that wheatgrass may ease the symptoms of ulcerative colitis although further work needs to be undertaken.

Safety: Side-effects include nausea, vomiting and constipation and anorexia has been reported as a longer term complication: contraindicated in susceptible people.

### Bibliography

Ben-Arye E, Golden E, Wengrower D et al 2002 Wheat grass juice in the treatment of active distal ulcerative colitis a randomized double-blind placebo-controlled trial. Scandinavian Journal of Gastroenterology 4:444–449

*Cramp bark* (Viburnum opulus) *(also known as European cranberry bush, Guelder rose, High bush cranberry, Snowball bush)*

Traditional uses:   As its name suggests, cramp bark is traditionally used for cramps, including menstrual pain, muscular pain and cramps in pregnancy. Orally, it is used for spasmodic urinary conditions and as a diuretic, for infection, nervous disorders and as a sedative.

Principal constituents:   Scopoletin and viopudial have been identified, which, *in vitro*, appear to have smooth muscle antispasmodic effects. Other constituents include bitters, valerianic acid, salicosides, tannin and resin.

Evidence:   There is accumulating evidence of the antispasmodic effects of cramp bark.

Safety:   Concomitant use with diuretic drugs and other herbs is contraindicated. Bradycardia, hypotension and reduced myocardial contractility have been attributed to the viopudial content.

Bibliography

Nicholson J A, Darby T D, Jarboe C H 1972 Viopudial, a hypotensive and smooth muscle antispasmodic from Viburnum opulus. Proceedings of the Society for Experimental Biology and Medicine 140:457–461

Zayachkivska O S, Gzhegotsky M R, Terletska O I et al 2006 Influence of Viburnum opulus proanthocyanidins on stress-induced gastrointestinal mucosal damage. Journal of Physiology and Pharmacology 57(Suppl 5):155–167

*Cranberry* (Vaccinium macrocarpon)

Traditional uses:   Cranberry is well known as a remedy for preventing and treating urinary tract infections and has also been used for haematological disorders, gastric ailments, hepatic conditions and anorexia.

Principal constituents:   acids, carbohydrates, phenolics.

Evidence:   Studies indicate inhibition of *Escherichia coli* and *Enterococcus faecalis* in urinary tract infections but tests suggest that daily consumption of the unsweetened juice is required to prevent infection.

Safety:   Sugar free preparations should be used to avoid aggravation of urinary symptoms. Patients should not use cranberry juice as the sole remedy for urinary tract infections, when antibiotics are indicated. Do not confuse with cramp bark, sometimes known as European cranberry bush.

Bibliography

Cimolai N, Cimolai T 2007 Cranberry and the urinary tract. European Journal of Clinical and Microbiological Infectious Diseases 26(11):767–776

Dugoua J J, Seely D, Perri D et al 2008 Safety and efficacy of cranberry (Vaccinium macrocarpon) during pregnancy and lactation. Canadian Journal of Clinical Pharmacology 15(1):e80–e86

Gupta K, Chou M Y, Howell A 2007 Cranberry products inhibit adherence of p-fimbriated Escherichia coli to primary cultured bladder and vaginal epithelial cells. Journal of Urology 177(6):2357–2360

Jepson R G, Craig J C 2008 Cranberries for preventing urinary tract infections. Cochrane Database of Systematic Reviews(1): CD001321

McKay D L, Blumberg J B 2007 Cranberries (Vaccinium macrocarpon) and cardiovascular disease risk factors. Nutritional Review 65(11):490–502

Lavigne J P, Bourg G, Botto H et al 2007 Cranberry (Vaccinium macrocarpon) and urinary tract infections: study model and review of literature. Pathology Biology (Paris) 55(8–9):460–464

McKay D L, Blumberg J B 2007 Cranberries (Vaccinium macrocarpon) and cardiovascular disease risk factors. Nutritional Review 65(11):490–502

Neto C C 2007 Cranberry and blueberry: evidence for protective effects against cancer and vascular diseases. Molecular Nutritional Food Research 51(6): 652–664

Paeng C H, Sprague M, Jackevicius C A 2007 Interaction between warfarin and cranberry juice. Clinical Therapeutics 29(8):1730–1735

Wilson T, Singh A P, Vorsa N 2008 Human glycemic response and phenolic content of unsweetened cranberry juice. Journal of Medicinal Food 11(1):46–54

*Damiana* (Turnera diffusa) *(also known as Old woman's broom)*

Traditional uses:   Used for psycho-emotional sexual problems and for other emotional problems such as enuresis; also as a mild laxative.

Principal constituents:   flavonoids, terpenoids, saccharides and cyanogenic glycosides.

Evidence:   Non-clinical and clinical studies indicate that damiana is hypoglycaemic, a central nervous system depressant and antiinfective (*Escherichia coli, Proteus mirabilis, Pseudomonas aeruginosa* and *Staphylococcus aureus*).

Safety:   Large oral doses of damiana may cause spasmodic convulsions and paroxysms which presents with symptoms similar to rabies or strychnine poisoning. The hypoglycaemic action may theoretically interact with diabetic medication.

Bibliography

Alcaraz-Melendez L, Delgado-Rodriguez J, Real-Cosio S 2004 Analysis of essential oils from wild and micropropagated plants of damiana (Turnera diffusa). Fitoterapia 75:696–701

Arletti R, Benelli A, Cavazzuti E et al 1999 Stimulating property of Turnera diffusa and Pfaffia paniculata extracts on the sexual behavior of male rats. Psychopharmacology (Berl) 143:15–19

Ito T Y, Polan M L, Whipple B et al 2006 The enhancement of female sexual function with ArginMax, a nutritional supplement, among women differing in menopausal status. Journal of Sex Marital Therapy 32(5):369–378

Rowland D L, Tai W 2003 A review of plant-derived and herbal approaches to the treatment of sexual dysfunctions. Journal of Sex Marital Therapy 29(3):185–205

Zhao J, Pawar R S, Ali Z et al 2007 Phytochemical investigation of Turnera diffusa. Journal of Natural Products 70(2):289–292

*Dandelion* (Taraxacum officinale) *(also known as Lion's tooth, Fairy clock)*

Traditional uses:   Used as a digestive and hepatic tonic, laxative and diuretic, for gallstone and biliary conditions, chronic joint and skin problems.

Principal constituents:   bitter glycosides, sterols, tannins, rich in vitamins and minerals particularly potassium.

Evidence:   *In vitro* and animal studies indicate diuretic, anticoagulant, possible hypoglycaemic, antiinflammatory, increased bile secretion and anti-tumour properties.

Safety:   Contraindicated in people with clotting disorders or on anticoagulants, caution in diabetics.

Bibliography

Cuzzolin L, Zaffani S, Benoni G 2006 Safety implications regarding use of phytomedicines. European Journal of Clinical Pharmacology 62(1):37–42

Greenlee H, Atkinson C, Stanczyk F Z et al 2007 A pilot and feasibility study on the effects of naturopathic botanical and dietary interventions on sex steroid hormone metabolism in premenopausal women. Cancer Epidemiology, Biomarkers and Prevention 16(8):1601–1609

Jeon H J, Kang H J, Jung H J et al 2008 Antiinflammatory activity of Taraxacum officinale. Journal of Ethnopharmacology 115(1):82–88

Schütz K, Carle R, Schieber A 2006 Taraxacum – a review on its phytochemical and pharmacological profile. Journal of Ethnopharmacology 107(3):313–323

Sigstedt S C, Hooten C J, Callewaert M C et al 2008 Evaluation of aqueous extracts of Taraxacum officinale on growth and invasion of breast and prostate cancer cells. International Journal of Oncology 32(5):1085–1090

Sweeney B, Vora M, Ulbricht C et al 2005 Evidence-based systematic review of dandelion (Taraxacum officinale) by natural standard research collaboration. Journal of Herbal Pharmacotherapy 5(1):79–93

## Devil's claw (Harpagophytum procumbens) *(also known as Grapple plant, Wood spider)*

Traditional uses:  an antiinflammatory, analgesic, sedative and diuretic, for rheumatic and other joint pains, arteriosclerosis, allergies, headaches, intrapartum difficulties, renal and hepatic disorders and topically for skin conditions.

Principal constituents:  harpagoside, phenols, flavonoids.

Evidence:  Animal studies and clinical trials indicate analgesic, anticoagulant, hypoglycaemic, cardioactive, antiarrhythmic and possible antiinflammatory properties. Clinical studies indicate its possible value in low back pain and osteoarthritis.

Safety:  Side-effects include nausea, vomiting, diarrhoea, skin irritation and severe headaches. Contraindicated in people with clotting disorders or on anticoagulant medication. Caution in any cardiac pathology. Increases stomach acid and may decrease the effectiveness of antacids; contraindicated in patients with gastric or duodenal ulcers.

Bibliography

Brien S, Lewith G T, McGregor G 2006 Devil's claw (Harpagophytum procumbens) as a treatment for osteoarthritis: a review of efficacy and safety. Journal of Alternative and Complementary Medicine 12(10):981–993

Denner S S 2007 A review of the efficacy and safety of devil's claw for pain associated with degenerative musculoskeletal diseases, rheumatoid and osteoarthritis. Holistic Nurse Practice 21(4):203–207

Grant L, McBean D E, Fyfe L et al 2007 A review of the biological and potential therapeutic actions of Harpagophytum procumbens. Phytotherapy Research 21(3):199–209

Izzo A A, Di Carlo G, Borrelli F et al 2005 Cardiovascular pharmacotherapy and herbal medicines: the risk of drug interaction. International Journal of Cardiology 98(1):1–14

Vlachojannis J, Roufogalis B D, Chrubasik S 2008 Systematic review on the safety of Harpagophytum preparations for osteoarthritic and low back pain. Phytotherapy Research 22(2):149–152

Warnock M, McBean D, Suter A et al 2007 Effectiveness and safety of Devil's claw tablets in patients with general rheumatic disorders. Phytotherapy Research 21(12):1228–1233

*Drosera* (Drosera rotundifolia) *(also known as Sundew)*

Traditional uses: as an antispasmodic, demulcent and expectorant, used for asthma, respiratory tract infections, gastric ulceration.

Principal constituents: flavonoids, quinines.

Evidence: *In vitro* and animal studies indicate: antispasmodic, antimicrobial (v. *staphylococcus, streptococcus* and *pneumococcus*) and anti-tussive properties.

Safety: No information regarding safety or evidence of contraindications was found.

### Bibliography

Krenn L, Beyer G, Pertz H H et al 2004 In vitro antispasmodic and antiinflammatory effects of Drosera rotundifolia. Arzneimittelforschung 54(7):402–405

Melzig M F, Pertz H H, Krenn L 2001 Antiinflammatory and spasmolytic activity of extracts from Droserae herba. Phytomedicine 8(3):225–229

Murali P M, Rajasekaran S, Paramesh P et al 2006 Plant-based formulation in the management of chronic obstructive pulmonary disease: a randomized double-blind study. Respiratory Medicine 100(1):39–45

Paper D H, Karall E, Kremser M et al 2005 Comparison of the antiinflammatory effects of Drosera rotundifolia and Drosera madagascariensis in the HET-CAM assay. Phytotherapy Research 19(4):323–326

*Echinacea* (Echinacea augustifolia) *(also known as Cone flower)*

Traditional uses: to treat the common cold, catarrh, tonsillitis and other upper respiratory tract infections, acne, as well as skin infections, wound healing, urinary tract infections. Many people use it as a means of preventing winter colds.

Principal constituents: alkaloids, carbohydrates, glycosides, terpenoids, glycol-proteins, essential oils.

Evidence: Studies have demonstrated immunostimulant activity, phagocyte enhancement, antiinflammatory and antibacterial (*Escherichia coli, Pseudomonas aeruginosa, Staphylococcus aureus*) properties.

Safety: As with all herbal remedies, echinacea should only be taken as required and should not be taken for longer than three months at a time; it is inappropriate for people to self-medicate in the long term. Side-effects include nausea, vomiting, abdominal pain, diarrhoea, allergic reactions including a burning sensation and tingling and numbness of the tongue, headache, dizziness, insomnia, disorientation and anaphylaxis.

Bibliography

Birt D F, Widrlechner M P, Lalone C A 2008 Echinacea in infection. American Journal of Clinical Nutrition 87(2):488S–492S

Gurley B J, Swain A, Hubbard M A et al 2008 Clinical assessment of CYP2D6-mediated herb-drug interactions in humans: effects of milk thistle, black cohosh, goldenseal, kava kava, St. John's wort and Echinacea. Molecular Nutrition and Food Research 52(7):755–763

Hellum B H, Nilsen O G 2007 The in vitro inhibitory potential of trade herbal products on human CYP2D6-mediated metabolism and the influence of ethanol. Basic Clinical Pharmacology and Toxicology 101(5):350–358

Kocaman O, Hulagu S, Senturk O 2008 Echinacea-induced severe acute hepatitis with features of cholestatic autoimmune hepatitis. European Journal of Internal Medicine 19(2):148

O'Neil J, Hughes S, Lourie A et al 2008 Effects of echinacea on the frequency of upper respiratory tract symptoms: a randomized, double-blind, placebo-controlled trial. Annals of Allergy, Asthma and Immunology 100(4):384–388

Saunders P R, Smith F, Schusky R W 2007 Echinacea purpurea L. in children: safety, tolerability, compliance and clinical effectiveness in upper respiratory tract infections. Canadian Journal of Physiology Pharmacology 85(11):1195–1199

Tierra M 2007 Echinacea: an effective alternative to antibiotics. Journal of Herbal Pharmacotherapy 7(2):79–89

## Elder (Sambucus nigra)

Traditional uses:   as an expectorant, diuretic, antiinflammatory and for fever, respiratory tract infections and catarrh.

Principal constituents:   volatile oil, flavonoids, tannins, mucilage.

Evidence:   Studies indicate diuretic and laxative, antiinflammatory, hypoglycaemic, antispasmodic and antiviral (influenza types A and B and herpes simplex type 1) properties.

Safety:   Caution regarding concurrent medication, herbs and supplements with similar therapeutic actions, in particular other herbs with diuretic properties which may potentiate the effects; increased effects have also been noted when combined with antioxidants such as vitamin C.

Bibliography

Gorchakova T V, Suprun I V, Sobenin I A et al 2007 Use of natural products in anticytokine therapy. Bulletin of Experimental Biology and Medicine 143(3):316–319

Gray A M, Abdel-Wahab Y H, Flatt P R 2000 The traditional plant treatment, Sambucus nigra (elder), exhibits insulin-like and insulin-releasing actions in vitro. Journal of Nutrition 130(1):15–20

Zakay-Rones Z, Thom E, Wollan T et al 2004 Randomized study of the efficacy and safety of oral elderberry extract in the treatment of influenza A and B virus infections. Journal of International Medical Research 32(2):132–140

## *Elecampane* (Inula helenium) *(also known as Horse heal, Scabwort)*

Traditional uses:   Used as a stimulant, expectorant, digestive tonic, relaxant and for bronchial and pulmonary conditions.

Principal constituents:   volatile oil including camphor, saponins, mucilage, carbohydrates, terpenoids.

Evidence:   Trials indicate antitussive, sedative and antibacterial properties, as well as an effect on angina and myocardial conditions.

Safety:   Caution with concurrent sedation and analgesics containing codeine; and in patients hypersensitive to chrysanthemums, daisies and marigolds. May reduce the effectiveness of anti-diabetic medication.

Bibliography

Aberer W 2008 Contact allergy and medicinal herbs. Journal of the German Society of Dermatology 6(1):15–24

Cantrell C L, Abate L, Fronczek F R et al 1999 Antimycobacterial eudesmanolides from Inula helenium and Rudbeckia subtomentosa. Planta Medica 65(4):351–355

Paulsen E 2002 Contact sensitization from Compositae-containing herbal remedies and cosmetics. Contact Dermatitis 47(4):189–198

## *Ephedra* (Ephedraceae) *(also known as Ma huang, Natural ecstasy)*

Traditional uses:   Commonly used as a peripheral dilator, for allergic rhinitis, nasal congestion and as a bronchial relaxant. It is also used as a central nervous system stimulant and to enhance myocardial contraction.

Principal Constituents:   ephedrine, methyl ephedrine and norephedrine, volatile oil, tannins, flavonoids.

Evidence:   Trials indicate that ephedra is inflammatory, a stimulant to the central nervous system, a bronchial relaxant, antibacterial (*Staphylococcus aureus*), hyperglycaemic and hypertensive.

Safety:   Ephedra is a cardiac stimulant and may interfere with the action of cardiac glycosides, may cause tachycardia, cardiac arrhythmias and cardiomyopathy. It may decrease the effectiveness of anti-hypertensive and anti-diabetic therapy. Caution with caffeine-containing drinks. Contraindicated in patients on monoamine oxidase inhibitors.

### Bibliography

Berman J A, Setty A, Steiner M J 2006 Complicated hypertension related to the abuse of ephedrine and caffeine alkaloids. Journal of Addictive Diseases 25(3):45–48

Caron M F, Dore D D, Min B et al 2006 Electrocardiographic and blood pressure effects of the ephedra-containing TrimSpa thermogenic herbal compound in healthy volunteers. Pharmacotherapy 26(9):1241–1246

Chitturi S, Farrell G C 2008 Hepatotoxic slimming aids and other herbal hepatotoxins. Journal of Gastroenterology and Hepatology 23(3):366–373

Fleming R M 2007 The effect of ephedra and high fat dieting: a cause for concern! A case report. Angiology 58(1):102–105

Singh A, Rajeev A G, Dohrmann M L 2008 Cardiomyopathy associated with ephedra-containing nutritional supplements. Congestive Heart Failure 14(2):89–90.

## *Euphorbia* (Euphorbia hirta) *(also known as Snakeweed)*

Traditional uses: Commonly used for respiratory tract infections, asthma, catarrh and laryngeal spasm, but also used in Indian medicine for worms, dysentery, gonorrhoea and digestive problems.

Principal constituents: flavonoids, terpenoids, sugars, choline, resins and alkaloids.

Evidence: Euphorbia has been shown to be antispasmodic, antihistaminic and antibacterial (Gram-positive and Gram-negative).

Safety: Side-effects include nausea, vomiting, dermatitis and gastric irritation, including exacerbation of existing gastrointestinal conditions.

### Bibliography

Chaabi M, Freund-Michel V, Frossard N 2007 Anti-proliferative effect of Euphorbia stenoclada in human airway smooth muscle cells in culture. Journal of Ethnopharmacology 109(1):134–139

Hore S K, Ahuja V, Mehta G 2006 Effect of aqueous Euphorbia hirta leaf extract on gastrointestinal motility. Fitoterapia 77(1):35–38

Ndip R N, Malange Tarkang A E, Mbullah S M et al 2007 In vitro anti-Helicobacter pylori activity of extracts of selected medicinal plants from North West Cameroon. Journal of Ethnopharmacology 114(3):452–457

Singh G D, Kaiser P, Youssouf M S et al 2006 Inhibition of early and late phase allergic reactions by Euphorbia hirta L. Phytotherapy Research 20(4):316–321

Sudhakar M, Rao Ch V, Rao P M et al 2006 Antimicrobial activity of Caesalpinia pulcherrima, Euphorbia hirta and Asystasia gangeticum. Fitoterapia 77(5):378–380

Youssouf M S, Kaiser P, Tahir M et al 2007 Anti-anaphylactic effect of Euphorbia hirta. Fitoterapia 78(7–8):535–539

## Fenugreek (Trigonella foenum-graecum)

Traditional uses:   Used in medicinal systems in India and the Indian sub-continent, as a digestive tonic, for gastric inflammation, dyspepsia and anorexia; it is also thought to promote lactation and is used topically for skin inflammations.

Principal constituents:   steroidal saponins, mucilages, volatile oils, alkaloids, coumarins and lipids.

Evidence:   *In vitro* animal studies and clinical trials indicate hypoglycaemic, diuretic, cholesterol- and triglyceride-reducing properties.

Safety:   Side-effects include diarrhoea, heartburn and abdominal discomfort, allergic and anaphylactic reactions; large doses may cause hypoglycaemia. People who are allergic to soy beans, chick peas, peanuts and green peas may be more at risk of allergic reaction due to cross-reactivity. It is considered unsafe in children and should be avoided by pregnant women, except as a culinary additive, as the neonate may be born with an unusual body odour similar to maple syrup urine disease. There have been isolated reports of loss of consciousness in children who have consumed the tea. There is a moderate theoretical risk of interaction with anticoagulant and antiplatelet drugs, as well as with diabetic medication.

### Bibliography

Ali-Shtayeh M S, Jamous R M, Al-Shafie J H et al 2008 Traditional knowledge of wild edible plants used in Palestine (Northern West Bank): a comparative study. Journal of ethnobiology and Ethnomedicine 4(1):13

Arayne M S, Sultana N, Mirza A Z et al 2007 In vitro hypoglycemic activity of methanolic extract of some indigenous plants. Pakistan Journal of Pharmaceutical Sciences 20(4):268–273

Izzo A A, Di Carlo G, Borrelli F et al 2005 Cardiovascular pharmacotherapy and herbal medicines: the risk of drug interaction. International Journal of Cardiology 98(1):1–14

Modak M, Dixit P, Londhe J et al 2007 Indian herbs and herbal drugs used for the treatment of diabetes. Journal of Clinical Biochemistry and Nutrition 40(3):163–173

Sewell A C, Mosandl A, Böhles H 1999 False diagnosis of maple syrup urine disease owing to ingestion of herbal tea. New England Journal of Medicine 341(10):769

Vijayakumar M V, Bhat M K 2008 Hypoglycemic effect of a novel dialysed fenugreek seeds extract is sustainable and is mediated, in part, by the activation of hepatic enzymes. Phytotherapy Research 22(4):500–505

## Feverfew (Tanacetum parthenium) *(also known as Bachelor's buttons, Featherwort, Midsummer daisy)*

Traditional uses: as an antiinflammatory, vasodilator, uterine stimulant, relaxant, digestive stimulant, for migraine, headaches, eczema, arthritis, vertigo, tinnitus and congestive dysmenorrhoea.

Principal constituents: terpenoids, volatile oils, flavonoids, tannins, monoterpene and sesquiterpene components, melatonin.

Evidence: Trials indicate antiinflammatory and anticoagulant properties and support its use in migraine prophylaxis.

Safety: Side-effects include gastrointestinal complaints, headaches, joint pain and weight gain. Topical use can cause dermatitis. There is a moderate risk of interaction with anticoagulants, those with clotting defects should avoid using it.

### Bibliography

Diener H C, Pfaffenrath V, Schnitker J et al 2005 Efficacy and safety of 6.25 mg t.i.d. feverfew CO2-extract (MIG-99) in migraine prevention – a randomized, double-blind, multicentre, placebo-controlled study. Cephalalgia 25:1031–1041

Eichenfield L F, Fowler J F Jr, Rigel D S et al 2007 Natural advances in eczema care. Cutis 80(Suppl):2–16

Ernst E, Pittler M H 2000 The efficacy and safety of feverfew (Tanacetum parthenium L.): an update of a systematic review. Public Health and Nutrition 3:509–514

Evans R W, Taylor F R 2006 'Natural' or alternative medications for migraine prevention. Headache 46(6):1012–1018

Maizels M, Blumenfeld A, Burchette R 2004 A combination of riboflavin, magnesium and feverfew for migraine prophylaxis: a randomized trial. Headache 44(9):885–890

Pfaffenrath V, Diener H C, Fischer M et al 2002 The efficacy and safety of Tanacetum parthenium (feverfew) in migraine prophylaxis – a double-blind, multicentre, randomized placebo-controlled dose-response study. Cephalalgia 22:523–532

Schürks M, Diener H C, Goadsby P 2008 Update on the prophylaxis of migraine. Current Treatment Options in Neurology 10(1):20–29

## Flax (Linum usitatissimum) *(also known as Linseed, Flaxseed)*

Traditional uses:  as a laxative for chronic constipation, disorders of the colon, irritable bowel syndrome and externally as a poultice for local areas of inflammation.

Principal constituents:  unsaturated fatty acids, soluble fibre, linolenic, linoleic and oleic acids.

Evidence:  *In vitro* and animal studies indicate hypocholesterolaemic and hypotensive properties. Clinical trials indicate musculoskeletal improvements. May have some benefit for women with perimenopausal symptoms.

Safety:  Contraindicated in patients with or at risk of prostate cancer and those with suspected or actual paralytic ileus. Side-effects are similar to other preparations used for gastrointestinal conditions, including diarrhoea, bloating abdominal and flatulence. Anaphylactic shock has been reported.

### Bibliography

Brooks J D, Ward W E, Lewis J E et al 2004 Supplementation with flaxseed alters estrogen metabolism in postmenopausal women to a greater extent than does supplementation with an equal amount of soy. American Journal of Clinical Nutrition 79:318–325

Chilibeck P D, Cornish S M 2008 Effect of estrogenic compounds (estrogen or phytoestrogens) combined with exercise on bone and muscle mass in older individuals. Applied Physiology Nutrition and Metabolism 33(1):200–212

Demark-Wahnefried W, Robertson C N, Walther P J et al 2004 Pilot study to explore effects of low-fat, flaxseed-supplemented diet on proliferation of benign prostatic epithelium and prostate-specific antigen. Urology 63:900–904

Dodin S, Lemay A, Jacques H et al 2005 The effects of flaxseed dietary supplement on lipid profile, bone mineral density and symptoms in menopausal women: a randomized, double-blind, wheat germ placebo-controlled clinical trial. Journal of Clinical Endocrinology and Metabolism 90:1390–1397

Doughman S D, Krupanidhi S, Sanjeevi C B 2007 Omega-3 fatty acids for nutrition and medicine: considering microalgae oil as a vegetarian source of EPA and DHA. Current Diabetes Review 3(3):198–203

Haggans C J, Travelli E J, Thomas W et al 2000 The effect of flaxseed and wheat bran consumption on urinary estrogen metabolites in premenopausal women. Cancer Epidemiology, Biomarkers and Prevention 9:719–725

Knudsen V K, Hansen H S, Osterdal M L 2006 Fish oil in various doses or flax oil in pregnancy and timing of spontaneous delivery: a randomised controlled trial. British Journal of Obstetrics and Gynaecology 113(5):536–543

Leon F, Rodriguez M, Cuevas M 2003 Anaphylaxis to Linum. Allergologia et immunopathologia 31:47–49

Lucas E A, Wild R D, Hammond L J et al 2002 Flaxseed improves lipid profile without altering biomarkers of bone metabolism in postmenopausal women. Journal of Clinical Endocrinology and Metabolism 87:1527–1532

Schabath M B, Hernandez L M, Wu X et al 2005 Dietary phytoestrogens and lung cancer risk. Journal of the American Medical Association 294:1493–1504

Stuglin C, Prasad K 2005 Effect of flaxseed consumption on blood pressure, serum lipids, hemopoietic system and liver and kidney enzymes in healthy humans. Journal of Cardiovascular Pharmacology and Therapeutics 10(1):23–27

## Garlic (Allium sativum)

Traditional uses: Used for its purported antimicrobial, hypocholesterolaemic, vasodilatory, antihistaminic, antispasmodic and anticoagulant properties.

Principal constituents: allicin, potassium, zinc, proteins, vitamins and minerals, lipids and prostaglandins.

Evidence: *In vitro* animal studies and clinical trials indicate hypocholesterolaemic, anti-atherosclerotic, anticoagulant action and anti-hypertensive, antimicrobial (*Staphylococcus aureus, Staphylococcus faecalis, Candida albicans, Proteus, Salmonella, Escherichia coli*) properties.

Safety: Garlic may increase the risk of bleeding in patients with bleeding disorders or taking anticoagulants including aspirin and NSAIDs. Caution in diabetes as garlic may affect blood glucose levels.

### Bibliography

Borrelli F, Capasso R, Izzo A A 2007 Garlic (Allium sativum L.): adverse effects and drug interactions in humans. Molecular Nutrition Food Research 51(11): 1386–1397

Izzo A A, Di Carlo G, Borrelli F et al 2005 Cardiovascular pharmacotherapy and herbal medicines: the risk of drug interaction. International Journal of Cardiology 98(1):1–14

Liu C T, Sheen L Y, Lii C K 2007 Does garlic have a role as an antidiabetic agent? Molecular Nutrition and Food Research 51(11):1353–1364

Morihara N, Nishihama T, Ushijima M et al 2007 Garlic as an anti-fatigue agent. Molecular Nutrition and Food Research 51(11):1329–1334

Ngo S N, Williams D B, Cobiac L et al 2007 Does garlic reduce risk of colorectal cancer? A systematic review. Journal of Nutrition 137(10):2264–2269

Scharbert G, Kalb M L, Duris M 2007 Garlic at dietary doses does not impair platelet function. Anesthetic Analgesia 105(5):1214–1218

## Gentian (Gentiana lutea) *(also known as Bitterroot, Bitterwort)*

Traditional uses:   for gastrointestinal conditions, gastric inflammation, hepatic and gall bladder disease; topically it is used for wound healing.

Principal constituents:   bitter glycosides, alkaloids and flavonoids.

Evidence:   *In vitro* and animal studies indicate antiinflammatory, antifungal, hypotensive, choleretic properties and stimulation of gastric juices. Clinical studies indicate stimulation of gastric juices.

Safety:   Caution regarding concurrent medication, herbs and supplements with diuretic and anti-hypertensive effects, which may potentiate the effects.

### Bibliography

Baragatti B, Calderone V, Testai L et al 2002 Vasodilator activity of crude methanolic extract of Gentiana kokiana Perr. et Song. (Gentianaceae). Journal of Ethnopharmacology 79:369–372

Haraguchi H, Tanaka Y, Kabbash A et al 2004 Monoamine oxidase inhibitors from Gentiana lutea. Phytochemistry 65:2255–2260

Uncini Manganelli R E, Chericoni S, Baragatti B 2000 Ethnopharmacobotany in Tuscany: plants used as anti-hypertensives. Fitoterapia 71:S95–100

## Ginger (Zingiber officinale)

Traditional uses:    as a circulatory stimulant and vasodilator, pulmonary antiseptic, antispasmodic, antiemetic and used in treatment of inflammatory conditions such as osteo- and rheumatoid arthritis.

Principal constituents: volatile oil, phenols, gingerols, lipids, vitamins and minerals.

Evidence:   *In vitro* animal studies and clinical trials indicate: anti-inflammatory, antiplatelet properties and anti-emetic activity. There is also growing evidence of the anticoagulant properties of ginger.

Safety:   Caution regarding the increased risk of bleeding in patients with bleeding disorders or taking anticoagulants including aspirin and non-steroidal antiinflammatories. Prolonged continual use of more than 1 g/day for 3 weeks or more should be discouraged and patients who use ginger, particularly pregnant women requiring its anti-emetic properties, should have their clotting factors assessed. Patients with any cardiovascular pathology should avoid ginger, which may also diminish the effect of anti-hypertensive therapy. Side-effects include heartburn and hot flushes.

## Bibliography

Chrubasik S, Pittler M H, Roufogalis B D 2005 Zingiberis rhizoma: a comprehensive review on the ginger effect and efficacy profiles. Phytomedicine 12(9):684–701

Ensiyeh J, Sakineh M A 2008 Comparing ginger and vitamin B6 for the treatment of nausea and vomiting in pregnancy: a randomised controlled trial. Midwifery 11 Feb

Ghayur M N, Gilani A H, Janssen L J 2008 Ginger attenuates acetylcholine-induced contraction and Ca2+ signalling in murine airway smooth muscle cells. Canadian Journal of Physiology and Pharmacology 86(5):264–271

Gregory P J, Sperry M, Wilson A F 2008 Dietary supplements for osteoarthritis. American Family Physician 77(2):177–184

Hoffman T 2007 Ginger: an ancient remedy and modern miracle drug. Hawaii Medical Journal 66(12):326–327

Minghetti P, Sosa S, Cilurzo F 2007 Evaluation of the topical antiinflammatory activity of ginger dry extracts from solutions and plasters. Planta Medica 73(15): 1525–1530

Nanthakomon T, Pongrojpaw D 2006 The efficacy of ginger in prevention of postoperative nausea and vomiting after major gynecologic surgery. Journal of the Medical Association Thailand 89(Suppl 4):S130–S136

Nicoll R, Henein M Y 2007 Ginger (Zingiber officinale Roscoe): a hot remedy for cardiovascular disease? International Journal of Cardiology 23 Nov

Rhode J, Fogoros S, Zick S et al 2–7 Ginger inhibits cell growth and modulates angiogenic factors in ovarian cancer cells. BMC Complementary and Alternative Medicine 7:44

Shalansky S, Lynd L, Richardson K et al 2007 Risk of warfarin-related bleeding events and supratherapeutic international normalized ratios associated with complementary and alternative medicine: a longitudinal analysis. Pharmacotherapy 27(9):1237–1247

Wu K L, Rayner C K, Chuah S K et al 2008 Effects of ginger on gastric emptying and motility in healthy humans. European Journal of Gastroenterology and Hepatology 20(5):436–440

*Ginkgo biloba* (Ginkgo biloba)

Traditional uses: Historically used for asthma and cardiovascular disorders such as cardiac arrhythmias, now used for cognitive deficiency, intermittent claudication, vertigo and tinnitus.

Principal constituents: amino acids, flavonoids, terpenoids.

Evidence: *In vitro* animal studies and clinical trials indicate cognitive, learning and memory enhancement, cardiovascular and anticoagulant properties.

Safety: Caution regarding concurrent medication, herbs and supplements with similar therapeutic action. Decreases the seizure threshold of anticonvulsant medication.

Bibliography

Bone K M 2008 Potential interaction of Ginkgo biloba leaf with antiplatelet or anticoagulant drugs: what is the evidence? Molecular Nutrition Food Research 23 Jan

Dodge H H, Zitzelberger T, Oken B S 2008 A randomized placebo-controlled trial of ginkgo biloba for the prevention of cognitive decline. Neurology 27 Feb

Hellum B H, Nilsen O G 2007 The in vitro inhibitory potential of trade herbal products on human CYP2D6-mediated metabolism and the influence of ethanol. Basic Clinical Pharmacology Toxicology 101(5):350–358

Izzo A A, Di Carlo G, Borrelli F et al 2005 Cardiovascular pharmacotherapy and herbal medicines: the risk of drug interaction. International Journal of Cardiology 98(1):1–14

Mahadevan S, Park Y 2008 Multifaceted therapeutic benefits of Ginkgo biloba L: chemistry, efficacy, safety and uses. Journal of Food Science 73(1):R14–R19

Meston C M, Rellini A H, Telch M J 2008 Short- and long-term effects of Ginkgo biloba extract on sexual dysfunction in women. Archives in Sexual Behavior 37(4):530–547

*Ginseng* (Ginseng panax) *(Chinese ginseng, Asiatic ginseng)*

Traditional uses: as an adaptogen by acting on the adrenal cortex and stimulating or relaxing the nervous system to restore emotional and physical balance and to improve well-being in degenerative conditions and old age.

Principal constituents: triterpenoid saponins, panax acid, glycosides, sterols and essential oil.

Evidence: Trials indicate hypoglycaemic, cardiovascular, antiviral, psychomotor enhancement, blood pressure normalization and asthma control properties. Appears to be antioxidant and anti-carcinogenic.

Safety: Caution with concurrent medication, herbs and supplements with similar therapeutic action and with steroid therapy. Contraindicated in psychiatric illness particularly, mania, schizophrenia, nervous tension, hyperactivity. Women may experience oestrogenic side-effects; contraindicated in pregnancy. People under 40 years of age should not take ginseng, nor should it be taken with stimulants including coffee or with antipsychotic drugs. Do not confuse with Siberian ginseng.

### Bibliography

Dasgupta A, Wu S, Actor J 2003 Effect of Asian and Siberian ginseng on serum digoxin measurement by five digoxin immunoassays. Significant variation in digoxin-like immunoreactivity among commercial ginsengs. American Journal of Clinical Pathology 119(2):298–303

Lee B, Yang C H, Hahm D H et al 2008 Inhibitory effects of ginseng total saponins on behavioral sensitization and dopamine release induced by cocaine. Biological and Pharmaceutical Bulletin 31(3):436–441

Seely D, Dugoua J J, Perri D 2008 Safety and efficacy of panax ginseng during pregnancy and lactation. Canadian Journal of Clinical Pharmacology 15(1):e87–e94

Sung W S, Lee D G 2008 In vitro candidacidal action of Korean red ginseng saponins against Candida albicans. Biological and Pharmaceutical Bulletin 31(1):139–142

Wang W, Rayburn E R, Hao M et al 2008 Experimental therapy of prostate cancer with novel natural product anti-cancer ginsenosides. Prostate 68(8):809–819

*Ginseng* (Ginseng eleutherococcus) *(Siberian ginseng)*

Traditional uses: to improve mental and physical stamina in extreme circumstances, also used for debility and depression.

Principal constituents: triterpenoid saponins, resin, starch, vitamin A.

Evidence: Studies indicate hypo/hyperglycaemic, central nervous system stimulating, cardiovascular, mental and physical enhancement properties.

Safety: Extreme caution in any cardiac pathology. Contraindicated in psychiatric illness, particularly mania, schizophrenia, nervous tension and hyperactivity. Caution in perimenopausal women and people under 40 years of age. It should not be taken with stimulants including coffee, nor with antipsychotic drugs; contraindicated with monoamine oxidase inhibitors. Do not confuse with Asian/Chinese ginseng.

Bibliography

Cicero A F, Derosa G, Brillante R et al 2004 Effects of Siberian ginseng (Eleutherococcus senticosus maxim.) on elderly quality of life: a randomized clinical trial. Archives of Gerontology and Geriatrics 9(Suppl):69–73

Dasgupta A, Wu S, Actor J et al 2003 Effect of Asian and Siberian ginseng on serum digoxin measurement by five digoxin immunoassays. Significant variation in digoxin-like immunoreactivity among commercial ginsengs. American Journal of Clinical Pathology 19(2):298–303

Hartz A J, Bentler S, Noyes R et al 2004 Randomized controlled trial of Siberian ginseng for chronic fatigue. Psychological Medicine 34(1):51–61

Izzo A A, Di Carlo G, Borrelli F et al 2005 Cardiovascular pharmacotherapy and herbal medicines: the risk of drug interaction. International Journal of Cardiology 98(1):1–14

## Goldenseal (Hydrastis canadensis) *(also known as Eye balm, Eye root)*

Traditional uses: as an astringent, digestive stimulant, healing herb for the gut wall and mucous membranes, used for postpartum haemorrhage, menorrhagia, gastritis, eczema, mouth and gastric ulcers, as a diuretic and laxative.

Principal constituents: alkaloids including berberine, volatile oil and resin.

Evidence: *In vitro* and animal studies indicate uterine stimulation, antihistamine, hypertensive and antimicrobial (*Staphylococcus, Streptococcus, Chlamydia aureus, Trichomonas vaginalis, Pseudomonas aeruginosa*) properties.

Safety: Possible emmenagogic and oxytocic effects make it theoretically unsafe in pregnancy, especially as berberine crosses the placenta and may be teratogenic. Contraindicated in neonates – berberine may cause kernicterus, via the breast milk. High doses/prolonged use may cause nausea, constipation, delirium, convulsions, paralysis, cardiac compromise, death. Vaginal douching with goldenseal may cause mucosal irritation and ulceration. Avoid in cardiovascular disease, hypertension, irritable bowel syndrome, Crohn's disease, ulcerative colitis. Possible interaction with anti-hypertensives, anticoagulants, barbiturates, sedatives, antacids.

Bibliography

Gurley B J, Swain A, Hubbard M A et al 2008 Clinical assessment of CYP2D6-mediated herb-drug interactions in humans: effects of milk thistle, black cohosh, goldenseal, kava kava, St. John's wort and Echinacea. Molecular Nutrition and Food Research 52(7):755–763

Palanisamy A, Haller C, Olson K R 2003 Photosensitivity reaction in a woman using an herbal supplement containing ginseng, goldenseal and bee pollen. Journal of Toxicology. Clinical Toxicology 41(6):865–867

Scazzocchio F, Cometa M F, Tomassini L et al 2001 Antibacterial activity of Hydrastis canadensis extract and its major isolated alkaloids. Planta Medica 67:561–564

## Green tea (Camellia sinensis)

Traditional uses:    popular in the east and becoming increasingly so in the west; it is traditionally used as an antibacterial, astringent, diuretic and stimulant and for the prevention of hypercholesterolemia and atherosclerosis.

Principal constituents:    polyphenols, tannins, flavonols, flavonoids, theobromine and theophylline.

Evidence:  Studies    indicate    cholesterol    lowering,    antibacterial (methicillin resistant *Staphylococcus aureus*) properties and inhibition of cell proliferation and tumour growth.

Safety:    Contains large doses of caffeine which may result in insomnia and cardiac arrhythmias; can inhibit anticoagulation therapy, significant source of vitamin K, can antagonize warfarin.

Bibliography

Antonello M, Montemurro D, Bolognesi M 2007 Prevention of hypertension, cardiovascular damage and endothelial dysfunction with green tea extracts. American Journal of Hypertension 20(12):1321–1328

Farris P 2007 Idebenone, green tea and Coffeeberry extract: new and innovative antioxidants. Dermatologic Therapy 20(5):322–329

Izzo A A, Di Carlo G, Borrelli F et al 2005 Cardiovascular pharmacotherapy and herbal medicines: the risk of drug interaction. International Journal of Cardiology 98(1):1–14

Venables M C, Hulston C J, Cox H R et al 2008 Green tea extract ingestion, fat oxidation and glucose tolerance in healthy humans. American Journal of Clinical Nutrition 87(3):778–784

Xu J, Wang J, Deng F 2008 Green tea extract and its major component epigallocatechin gallate inhibits hepatitis B virus in vitro. Antiviral Research 78(3):242–249

Zhang M, Zhao X, Zhang X et al 2008 Possible protective effect of green tea intake on risk of adult leukaemia. British Journal of Cancer 98(1):168–170

### Hawthorn (Crataegus laevigata) *(also known as Mayflower)*

Traditional uses:   as a cardiotonic, coronary and peripheral dilator, used for intermittent claudication, slowing and tonifying the myocardium and for hypertension.

Principal constituents: amines, flavonoid glycosides, saponins, tannins, trimethylamine.

Evidence:   Clinical trials indicate that hawthorn acts as an ACE inhibitor, beta-blocker and coronary artery dilator.

Safety:   Caution regarding concurrent medication, herbs and supplements with similar therapeutic actions. Caution with concurrent sedation and analgesics containing codeine. May potentiate cardiac glycosides, therefore caution in any cardiovascular pathology.

Bibliography

Chang W T, Dao J, Shao Z H 2005 Hawthorn: potential roles in cardiovascular disease. American Journal of Chinese Medicine 33(1):1–10

Pittler M H, Guo R, Ernst E 2008 Hawthorn extract for treating chronic heart failure. Cochrane Database of Systematic Reviews(1), CD005312

Walker A F, Marakis G, Simpson E et al 2006 Hypotensive effects of hawthorn for patients with diabetes taking prescription drugs: a randomised controlled trial. British Journal of General Practitioners 56(527):437–443

Zick S M, Blume A, Aaronson K D 2005 The prevalence and pattern of complementary and alternative supplement use in individuals with chronic heart failure. Journal of Cardiac Failure 11(8):586–589

### Hops (Humulus lupulus)

Traditional uses:   Long used as a sedative, antibacterial, anti-spasmodic, digestive tonic for insomnia, anxiety, restlessness, nervous dyspepsia and spastic constipation.

Principal constituents: volatile oil, bitter resin complex, tannins, asparagine, oestrogenic substances.

Evidence:   Trials indicate antispasmodic, antibacterial (*Candida*, *Staphylococcus aureus*) oestrogenic and sedative properties.

Safety:   Caution with concurrent sedation and analgesics containing codeine. Contraindicated in individuals suffering from depression. May interfere with tricyclic antidepressants, antipsychotics, benzodiazepines, oral hypoglycaemic agents, angiotensin II receptor antagonists, proton pump inhibitors, warfarin, non-steroidal antiinflammatories including aspirin, antihistamines and thyroid therapy. Caution in hormone sensitive conditions including women taking hormone replacement. May induce hyperglycaemia in diabetics and hypoglycaemia in non-diabetics.

Bibliography

Awad R, Levac D, Cybulska P 2007 Effects of traditionally used anxiolytic botanicals on enzymes of the gamma-aminobutyric acid (GABA) system. Canadian Journal of Physiology and Pharmacology 85(9):933–942

Heyerick A, Vervarcke S, Depypere H 2006 A first prospective, randomized, double-blind, placebo-controlled study on the use of a standardized hop extract to alleviate menopausal discomforts. Maturitas 54(2):164–175

Koetter U, Schrader E, Käufeler R et al 2007 A randomized, double blind, placebo-controlled, prospective clinical study to demonstrate clinical efficacy of a fixed valerian hops extract combination (Ze 91019) in patients suffering from non-organic sleep disorder. Phytotherapy Research 21(9):847–851

Morin C M, Koetter U, Bastien C et al 2005 Valerian-hops combination and diphenhydramine for treating insomnia: a randomized placebo-controlled clinical trial. Sleep 28(11):1465–1471

Natarajan P, Katta S, Andrei I et al 2008 Positive antibacterial co-action between hop (Humulus lupulus) constituents and selected antibiotics. Phytomedicine 15(3):194–201

Schiller H, Forster A, Vonhoff C et al 2006 Sedating effects of Humulus lupulus L. extracts. Phytomedicine 13(8):535–541

Zanoli P, Zavatti M 2008 Pharmacognostic and pharmacological profile of Humulus lupulus L. Ethnopharmacology 116(3):383–396

### Horse chestnut (Aesculus hippocastanum)

Traditional uses:  to reduce vasodilatation, antiinflammatory, used for varicose veins, haemorrhoids and phlebitis.

Principal constituents:  coumarins, flavonoids, tannins, saponins.

Evidence:  Studies suggest antiinflammatory, hypoglycaemic, anti-oedema and venous toning properties.

Safety:  Caution regarding concurrent medication, herbs and supplements with similar therapeutic. May increase risk of bleeding in patients with bleeding disorders or taking anticoagulants including aspirin and NSAIDs. Avoid in pregnancy, inflammatory bowel and haemorrhagic conditions, hepato-renal disorders and in those with a latex allergy. Avoid in diabetics. Saponin content may affect protein binding of some drugs. May cause gastric irritation, muscle twitching, paralysis, coma. Aesculin in raw seeds and bark may cause toxicity – European Union preparations are standardized for adults; avoid in children.

## Bibliography

Kahn S R 2006 Review: horse chestnut seed extract is effective for symptoms of chronic venous insufficiency. ACP Journal Club 145(1):20

Hellum B H, Nilsen O G 2007 The in vitro inhibitory potential of trade herbal products on human CYP2D6-mediated metabolism and the influence of ethanol. Basic Clinical Pharmacology and Toxicology 101(5):350–358

Hu J N, Zhu X M, Han L K et al 2008 Anti-obesity effects of escins extracted from the seeds of Aesculus turbinata BLUME (Hippocastanaceae). Chemical Pharmaceutical Bulletin (Tokyo) 56(1):12–16

Rathbun S W, Kirkpatrick A C 2007 Treatment of chronic venous insufficiency. Current Treatment Options in Cardiovascular Medicine 9(2):115–126

Suter A, Bommer S, Rechner J 2006 Treatment of patients with venous insufficiency with fresh plant horse chestnut seed extract: a review of 5 clinical studies. Advice Therapies 23(1):179–190

## Horsetail (Equisetum arvense) *(also known as Bottle brush, Shavegrass)*

Traditional uses:   as an astringent, strong diuretic used for oedema, urinary tract tonic.

Principal constituents:   silica, saponins, alkaloids, flavonoids.

Evidence:   *In vitro* animal and clinical studies indicate hypo-glycaemic, anticonvulsant, cardioactive and diuretic properties.

Safety:   Caution regarding concurrent medication, herbs and supplements with similar therapeutic action in particular other diuretic herbs which may potentiate the effects. May cause arrhythmias. May exacerbate effects of nicotine; caution with smokers and those using patches or gum.

## Bibliography

Correia H, Gonzalez-Paramas A, Amaral M T et al 2005 Characterisation of polyphenols by HPLC-PAD-ESI/MS and antioxidant activity in Equisetum telmateia. Phytochemical Analysis 16:380–387

Dos Santos J G Jr, Blanco M M, Do Monte F H et al 2005 Sedative and anticonvulsant effects of hydroalcoholic extract of Equisetum arvense. Fitoterapia 76:508–513

Revilla M C, Andrade-Cetto A, Islas S et al 2002 Hypoglycemic effect of Equisetum myriochaetum aerial parts on type 2 diabetic patients. Journal of Ethnopharmacology 81:117–120

## *Iscador* (Viscum album) *(also known as European mistletoe, All-heal, Devil's fuge, Mistletoe, Visci)*

Traditional uses:  First proposed as a treatment for cancer by Rudolph Steiner in 1920. An aqueous extract of mistletoe is fermented with the bacterium *Lactobacillus plantarum*), which is subsequently filtered out before administration. Subcutaneous injections are used for cancer treatments and for degenerative joint disease. It is also used orally to reduce chemotherapy and radiotherapy side-effects, as well as for hypertension, haemorrhage, haemorrhoids, convulsions, gout, depression and sleep disorders, headache and perimenopausal symptoms.

Principal constituents:  glycoprotein lectins, viscumin, viscotoxins, alkaloids and monoterpene glucosides.

Evidence:  There are several case reports regarding apparently successful use of Iscador in certain types of cancer, but formal trials do not support these examples for the majority of cancers. However, there is some emerging evidence that it may help in specific types of breast cancer, although the methodology of trials to date is not especially robust. It may have a part to play in the treatment of patients with hepatitis C, but further investigations are necessary.

Safety:  All parts of the mistletoe plant are toxic, but no serious side-effects were reported for Iscador. Some Australian mistletoe species are reported to extract toxic constituents from the host plant on which they grow therefore it is necessary to identify the host plant before using mistletoe. Not to be confused with American mistletoe. Side-effects from oral use include vomiting, diarrhoea, intestinal cramps, hepatitis, hypotension, uncontrollable eye movement, seizures, coma and death: dangers appear to be dose related, within fairly limited parameters and patients should be advised not to consume more than three mistletoe berries or two leaves and should refrain from self-administration. Subcutaneous adverse effects include pain at the injection site, pyrexia, headaches, angina, circulatory disturbance, allergic reaction and anaphylactic reactions. May interfere with the action of anti-hypertensive and immunostimulant medication and, specifically, with the herb hawthorn.

## Bibliography

Bar-Sela G, Goldberg H, Beck D 2006 Reducing malignant ascites accumulation by repeated intraperitoneal administrations of a Viscum album extract. Anticancer Research 26(1B):709–713

Bauer C, Oppel T, Rueff F et al 2005 Anaphylaxis to viscotoxins of mistletoe (Viscum album) extracts. Annals of Allergy, Asthma and Immunology 94: 86–89

Elsasser-Beile U, Leiber C, Wolf P et al 2005 Adjuvant intravesical treatment of superficial bladder cancer with a standardized mistletoe extract. Journal of Urology 174:76–79

Finall A I, McIntosh S A, Thompson W D 2006 Subcutaneous inflammation mimicking metastatic malignancy induced by injection of mistletoe extract. British Medical Journal 333:1293–1294

Grossarth-Maticek R, Ziegler R 2006 Prospective controlled cohort studies on long-term therapy of cervical cancer patients with a mistletoe preparation (Iscador). Forschende Komplementärmedizin 14(3):140–147

Grossarth-Maticek R, Ziegler R 2008 Randomized and non-randomized prospective controlled cohort studies in matched pair design for the long-term therapy of corpus uteri cancer patients with a mistletoe preparation (Iscador). European Journal of Medical Research 13(3):107–120

Heinzerling L, von Baehr V, Liebenthal C et al 2006 Immunologic effector mechanisms of a standardized mistletoe extract on the function of human monocytes and lymphocytes in vitro, ex vivo and in vivo. Journal of Clinical Immunology 26:347–359

Kirsch A 2007 Successful treatment of metastatic malignant melanoma with Viscum album extract (Iscador M). Journal of Alternative and Complementary Medicine 13(4):443–445

Steuer-Vogt M K, Bonkowsky V, Ambrosch P et al 2001 The effect of an adjuvant mistletoe treatment programme in resected head and neck cancer patients: a randomised controlled clinical trial. European Journal of Cancer 37: 23–31

Tusenius K J, Spoek J M, Kramers C W 2001 Iscador Qu for chronic hepatitis C: an exploratory study. Complementary Therapies in Medicine 9:12–16

## *Juniper berry* (Juniperus communis)

Traditional uses:  a popular remedy for cystitis, flatulence, colic; topically, for rheumatic pains.

Principal constituents:  flavonoids, acids, tannins, volatile oils, resins and sugars.

Evidence:   Trials have shown diuretic and antiinflammatory properties and transient hypertensive effects followed by a more prolonged hypotensive effect. May exacerbate seizures.

Safety:   Avoid in people with a compromised renal system or any renal or hepatic pathology. May exacerbate seizures. Avoid in pregnancy.

Bibliography

Filipowicz N, Kaminski M, Kurlenda J et al 2003 Antibacterial and antifungal activity of juniper berry oil and its selected components. Phytotherapy Research 7:227–231

Van Slambrouck S, Daniels A L, Hooten C J 2007 Effects of crude aqueous medicinal plant extracts on growth and invasion of breast cancer cells. Oncology Reports 17(6):1487–1492

Yarnell E 2002 Botanical medicines for the urinary tract. World Journal of Urology 20(5):285–293

*Kelp* (Laminaria digitata) *(also known as Seaweed, Bladderwrack)*

Traditional uses:   as a metabolic stimulant, thyroid restorative and antiinflammatory, for chronic joint pains, thyroid disorders and obesity.

Principal constituents:   mucilage, iodine, fucoidans, rich in vitamins and minerals.

Evidence:   Studies have demonstrated antioxidant effects and also suggest kelp may have a role in the management of perimenopausal symptoms; several case reports focus on the potential adverse effects.

Safety:   Caution regarding concurrent medication, herbs and supplements with similar therapeutic effects. May contain heavy metal contaminants. Advise patients not to consume excessive amounts as the iodine content may trigger thyroid problems; should be avoided by those with thyrotoxicosis.

Bibliography

Amster E, Tiwary A, Schenker M B 2007 Case report: potential arsenic toxicosis secondary to herbal kelp supplement. Environmental Health Perspectives 115(4):606–608

Clark C D, Bassett B, Burge M R 2003 Effects of kelp supplementation on thyroid function in euthyroid subjects. Endocrine Practice 9(5):363–369

Müssig K, Thamer C, Bares R 2006 Iodine-induced thyrotoxicosis after ingestion of kelp-containing tea. Journal of General Internal Medicine 21(6):C11–C14

Skibola C F 2004 The effect of Fucus vesiculosus, an edible brown seaweed, upon menstrual cycle length and hormonal status in three pre-menopausal women: a case report. BMC Complementary and Alternative Medicine 4:10

Yuan Y V, Walsh N A 2006 Antioxidant and antiproliferative activities of extracts from a variety of edible seaweeds. Food and Chemical Toxicology 44(7): 1144–1150

Zimmermann M, Delange F 2004 Iodine supplementation of pregnant women in Europe: a review and recommendations. European Journal of Clinical Nutrition 58(7):979–984

## Lady's mantle (Alchemilla vulgaris) *(also known as Bear's foot)*

Traditional uses: as an astringent both locally and systemically, used for correcting the menstrual cycle, general discharges and discharging wounds, enteritis and diarrhoea.

Principal constituents: tannins, flavonoids and glycoside.

Evidence: One animal study suggests a possible effect on blood pressure.

Safety: Lady's mantle has the theoretical possibility of causing hepatotoxicity, but reports are rare.

### Bibliography

Plotnikov M B, Aliev O I, Andreeva V Y et al 2006 Effect of Alchemilla vulgaris extract on the structure and function of erythrocyte membranes during experimental arterial hypertension. Bulletin of Experimental Biology and Medicine 141(6):708–711

## Lemon balm (Melissa officinalis)

Traditional uses: relaxant and sedative, used for calming central nervous system and digestive tensions.

Principal constituents: tannins, bitters, volatile oils, rosmarinic acid.

Evidence: Trials support the use of lemon balm as a relaxant and in the treatment of mild depression. Creams used locally for herpes appear to show significant improvement against placebo. There is some emerging evidence of its use in patients with HIV and other viral infections such as herpes simplex.

Safety: Caution with concurrent sedation and analgesics containing codeine.

Bibliography

Awad R, Levac D, Cybulska P 2007 Effects of traditionally used anxiolytic botanicals on enzymes of the gamma-aminobutyric acid (GABA) system. Canadian Journal of Physiology and Pharmacology 85(9):933–942

Geuenich S, Goffinet C, Venzke S et al 2008 Aqueous extracts from peppermint, sage and lemon balm leaves display potent anti-HIV-1 activity by increasing the virion density. Retrovirology 5:27

Kennedy D O, Little W, Haskell C F et al 2006 Anxiolytic effects of a combination of Melissa officinalis and Valeriana officinalis during laboratory induced stress. Phytotherapy Research 20(2):96–102

Kennedy D O, Wake G, Savelev S 2003 Modulation of mood and cognitive performance following acute administration of single doses of Melissa officinalis (Lemon balm) with human CNS nicotinic and muscarinic receptor-binding properties. Neuropsychopharmacology 28(10):1871–1881

Meolie A L, Rosen C, Kristo D; Clinical Practice Review Committee; American Academy of Sleep Medicine et al 2005 Oral nonprescription treatment for insomnia: an evaluation of products with limited evidence. Journal of Clinical Sleep Medicine 1(2):173–187

Müller S F, Klement S 2006 A combination of valerian and lemon balm is effective in the treatment of restlessness and dyssomnia in children. Phytomedicine 13(6):383–387

Sanchez-Medina A, Etheridge C J, Hawkes G E et al 2007 Comparison of rosmarinic acid content in commercial tinctures produced from fresh and dried lemon balm (Melissa officinalis). Journal of Pharmacy and Pharmaceutical Sciences 10(4):455–463

Ulbricht C, Brendler T, Gruenwald J; Natural Standard Research Collaboration 2005 Lemon balm (Melissa officinalis L.): an evidence-based systematic review by the Natural Standard Research Collaboration. Journal of Herbal Pharmacotherapy 5(4):71–114

## Lemon verbena (Aloysia triphylla; Lippia citriodora)

Traditional uses:   as an antispasmodic, antipyretic, sedative, used for asthma, colds, fever, flatulence and colic, diarrhoea and indigestion.

Principal constituents:   flavonoids and volatile oils.

Evidence:   There is little clinical evidence on the use of lemon verbena although studies investigating the antiinfective properties of essential plant oils occasionally include it amongst others. It may have antioxidant activity and has been shown to be effective against *Helicobacter pylori*.

Safety:   Orally lemon verbena may cause nephritis; contact dermatitis can occur with topical application.

Bibliography

Bilia A R, Giomi M, Innocenti M et al 2008 HPLC-DAD-ESI-MS analysis of the constituents of aqueous preparations of verbena and lemon verbena and evaluation of the antioxidant activity. Journal of Pharmaceutical and Biomedical Analysis 46(3):463–470

Ohno T, Kita M, Yamaoka Y et al 2003 Antimicrobial activity of essential oils against Helicobacter pylori. Helicobacter 8(3):207–215

## *Liquorice* (Glycyrrhiza glabra) *(also known as Sweet root)*

Traditional uses:   as a demulcent, expectorant, antiinflammatory, laxative and antispasmodic. Used for gastric ulcerations and inflammation.

Principal constituents:   glycosides, glycyrrhizin, triterpenoid saponins, flavonoids, bitters, volatile oil, coumarins, tannins.

Evidence: *In vitro* animal and clinical trials support the anti-inflammatory and demulcent, hormonal, hypertensive, electrolyte abnormalities, ACTH and diuretic effects; animal studies suggest a role in aiding memory, with possible future application to the management of Alzheimer's disease.

Safety:   Caution regarding concurrent medication, herbs and supplements with similar therapeutic actions; may increase the absorption rate of many drugs taken concomitantly including monamine oxidase inhibitors and corticosteroids. May decrease the effects of anti-hypertensive and diabetic therapy. Contraindicated in patients with any cardiovascular pathology. Poisoning can be insidious resulting in hypertension, hypokalaemia, sodium and water retention. Caution in hormone-sensitive conditions including hormone replacement therapy; avoid in pregnancy and lactation. Liquorice as a formal medication should only be used under the supervision of a qualified medical herbalist.

Bibliography

Cui Y M, Ao M Z, Li W et al 2008 Effect of glabridin from Glycyrrhiza glabra on learning and memory in mice. Planta Medica 74(4):377–380

Fiore C, Eisenhut M, Krausse R 2008 Antiviral effects of Glycyrrhiza species. Phytotherapy Research 22(2):141–148

Fukai T, Marumo A, Kaitou K et al 2002 Anti-Helicobacter pylori flavonoids from licorice extract. Life Sciences 71(12):1449–1463

Gupta V K, Fatima A, Faridi U et al 2008 Antimicrobial potential of Glycyrrhiza glabra roots. Journal of Ethnopharmacology 116(2):377–380

Mendes-Silva W, Assafim M, Ruta B 2003 Antithrombotic effect of Glycyrrhizin, a plant-derived thrombin inhibitor. Thrombosis Research 112(1–2):93–98

Nam C, Kim S, Sim Y et al 2003 Anti-acne effects of Oriental herb extracts: a novel screening method to select anti-acne agents. Skin Pharmacology Applied Skin Physiology 16(2):84–90

Saeedi M, Morteza-Semnani K, Ghoreishi M R 2003 The treatment of atopic dermatitis with licorice gel. Journal of Dermatological Treatment 14(3):153–157.

### *Lime blossom* (Tilia europea) *(also known as Linden blossom)*

Traditional uses:   as a peripheral vasodilator, sedative, antispasmodic, mild astringent and diuretic, for cardiovascular conditions with overlying tension and anxiety and as a hypotensive relaxant, particularly for children.

Principal constituents:   volatile oil, saponins, flavonoids, condensed tannins, mucilage.

Evidence:   *In vitro* studies have indicated antispasmodic effects and mild antifungal activity; the volatile oil has diuretic, sedative and antispasmodic effects.

Safety:   Caution regarding concurrent medication, herbs and supplements with similar therapeutic actions. Caution with concurrent sedation and analgesics containing codeine. May cause cardiac damage in patients with pre-existing disease; urticaria is possible with topical application.

#### Bibliography

No recent clinical literature found.

### *Lobelia* (Lobelia inflata) *(also known as Asthmaweed, Bladderpod, Indian tobacco, Pokeweed)*

Traditional uses: as a respiratory stimulant, antispasmodic, expectorant and emetic, used for chronic bronchitis and spasmodic asthma; also used topically for muscle inflammation, bruises, sprains, insect bites and ringworm.

Principal constituents:   alkaloids, fats, gum, resin, volatile oil, alpha lobeline.

Evidence:   Studies have demonstrated that alpha lobeline is similar in action to nicotine and affects peripheral circulation, the neuromuscular and central nervous systems. Alpha lobeline also stimulates respiration and acts as an expectorant when taken in small amounts, whereas larger amounts are emetic, purgative and diuretic effects. It is thought that, initially, lobeline stimulates the central nervous system, then depresses it, along with the respiratory system. Contemporary research suggests it may assist in reversing multidrug dependency in oncology patients; older studies theorize antidepressant properties, although this has not been demonstrated in any replicated studies.

Safety: Caution regarding concurrent medication, herbs and supplements with similar therapeutic action particularly CNS stimulants, including nicotine replacement therapy. Side-effects include nausea, vomiting, diarrhoea, coughing, dizziness and tremors, while overdose can lead to sweating, tachycardia, convulsions, hypothermia, hypotension, coma and death. Although traditionally used to aid smoking cessation, the US government prohibited lobeline in anti-smoking products in 1993.

Bibliography

Ma Y, Wink M 2008 Lobeline, a piperidine alkaloid from Lobelia can reverse P-gp dependent multidrug resistance in tumor cells. Phytomedicine 15(9):754–758

Mazur L J, De Ybarrondo L, Miller J et al 2001 Use of alternative and complementary therapies for pediatric asthma. Texas Medicine 97(6):64–68

## Marshmallow (Althaea officinalis; Althaea taurinensis)

Traditional uses: as a demulcent, bronchial dilator and diuretic, used for external wounds and burns, cystitis, gastritis and peptic ulceration.

Principal constituents: mucilage, asparagine, tannins, flavonoids, coumarins.

Evidence: There does not appear to be any recent clinical research specifically on marshmallow although the mucilage content has been proven. Mucilages are known to protect mucous membranes, suppress cough and have hypoglycemic effects, as well as being antimicrobial, spasmolytic, diuretic and wound-healing.

Safety: Caution regarding concurrent medication and herbs or supplements with similar effects. May interfere with the absorption of medication and may cause hypoglycaemia; avoid in diabetics on medication. Should not be confused with mallow and Chinese mallow.

Bibliography

Iauk L, Lo Bue A M, Milazzo I 2003 Antibacterial activity of medicinal plant extracts against periodontopathic bacteria. Phytotherapy Research 17(6):599–604

Kardosová A, Machová E 2006 Antioxidant activity of medicinal plant polysaccharides. Fitoterapia 77(5):367–373

Watt K, Christofi N, Young R 2007 The detection of antibacterial actions of whole herb tinctures using luminescent Escherichia coli. Phytotherapy Research 21(12):1193–1199

## Meadowsweet (Filipendula ulmaria) *(also known as Bridewort, Dropwort, Queen of the meadow)*

Traditional uses: for soothing and healing gastric mucosa, as a diuretic, antiseptic, antiinflammatory and antacid, used for urinary infections, oedema, gastritis.

Principal constituents: flavonoids, salicin, a plant salicylate, tannins, mucilages, volatile oils and heparin.

Evidence: Appears to have antioxidant and hepatoprotective effects; case reports highlight to potential adverse reactions to the salicylate content.

Safety: Caution regarding concurrent medication, herbs or supplements with similar effects. Meadowsweet potentiates the salicylate effect of other medications and herbs and specifically increases the risk of bleeding in patients with bleeding disorders or taking anticoagulants, aspirin and non-steroidal antiinflammatories. Contraindicated for asthmatics.

Bibliography

Abebe W 2002 Herbal medication: potential for adverse interactions with analgesic drugs. Journal of Clinical Pharmacy and Therapeutics 27(6):391–401

Heck A M, DeWitt B A, Lukes A L 2000 Potential interactions between alternative therapies and warfarin. American Journal of Health-system Pharmacy 57(13):1221–1227

Shilova I V, Zhavoronok T V, Suslov N I et al 2006 Hepatoprotective and antioxidant activity of meadowsweet extract during experimental toxic hepatitis. Bulletin of Experimental Biology and Medicine 142(2):216–218

## Milk thistle (Silybum marianum) *(also known as Silymarin, Lady's thistle, Marian thistle)*

Traditional uses: as a liver tonic and cleansing agent, for alcohol-related problems and for gall bladder disease.

Principal constituents: flavolignans, flavonoids, lipids, saponins.

Evidence: Clinical and non-clinical studies indicate liver cleansing/ healing properties with increased survival rates for alcoholic cirrhosis; there is some suggestion that milk thistle may offer protection against certain types of cancer and hepatitis C. It may also be effective as a hypoglycaemic agent in diabetes mellitus and appears, in combination with other herbs, to reduce dyspepsia.

Safety: Side-effects include diarrhoea, dyspepsia, flatulence, abdominal bloating, anorexia and allergic reactions such as pruritus, urticaria, eczema and anaphylaxis, particularly in those sensitive to chrysanthemums, marigolds and daisies. May interact with diazepam, warfarin and other similar drugs. It is thought that milk thistle may have oestrogenic effects therefore it should be avoided in those with hormone-sensitive conditions such as cancers, endometriosis and fibroids and is best avoided in pregnancy. Avoid confusion with Blessed thistle.

Bibliography

Agarwal R, Agarwal C, Ichikawa H 2006 Anticancer potential of silymarin: from bench to bed side. Anticancer Research 26(6B):4457–4498

Barve A, Khan R, Marsano L 2008 Treatment of alcoholic liver disease. Annals of Hepatology 7(1):5–15

Greenlee H, Abascal K, Yarnell E et al 2007 Clinical applications of Silybum marianum in oncology. Integrative Cancer Therapies 6(2):158–165

Gurley B J, Swain A, Hubbard M A 2008 Clinical assessment of CYP2D6-mediated herb-drug interactions in humans: effects of milk thistle, black cohosh, goldenseal, kava kava, St. John's wort and Echinacea. Molecular Nutrition and Food Research 52(7):755–763

Post-White J, Ladas E J, Kelly K M 2007 Advances in the use of milk thistle (Silybum marianum). Integrative Cancer Therapies 6(2):104–109

Ramasamy K, Agarwal R 2008 Multitargeted therapy of cancer by silymarin. Cancer Letters 8 May

Rambaldi A, Jacobs B P, Gluud C 2007 Milk thistle for alcoholic and/or hepatitis B or C virus liver diseases. Cochrane Database of Systematic Reviews(4): CD003620

Seeff L B, Curto T M, Szabo G; HALT-C Trial Group et al 2008 Herbal product use by persons enrolled in the hepatitis C antiviral long-term treatment against cirrhosis (HALT-C) trial. Hepatology 47(2):605–612

*American mistletoe* (Phoradendron leucarpum, Viscum leucarpum, Viscum flavescens, Phoradendron macrophyllum) *(also known as Eastern mistletoe, All-heal)*

Traditional uses:   as a smooth muscle stimulant, to increase blood pressure and to increase uterine contractions, particularly for abortion.

Principal constituents:   phoratoxins.

Evidence:   There is very little evidence on either the effectiveness or safety of American mistletoe, although it is possible that it may offer a role in treating breast cancer.

Safety:   Side-effects from ingestion include nausea, diarrhoea and vomiting leading to dehydration and hypovolaemic shock, bradycardia, hypertension, delirium, hallucinations, cardiac arrest and death. American mistletoe is probably unsafe for medicinal or recreational use and should be avoided. Avoid confusion with European mistletoe, Australian, Korean and New Zealand mistletoe. There is some evidence that the phoratoxins produce dose-dependent hyper- or hypotension, bradycardia, vasoconstriction, uterine and intestinal contractions and cardiac arrest, similar to the cardiotoxins from the venom of cobras. Avoid in pregnancy.

Bibliography

Johansson S, Gullbo J, Lindholm P et al 2003 Small, novel proteins from the mistletoe Phoradendron tomentosum exhibit highly selective cytotoxicity to human breast cancer cells. Cellular and Molecular Life Sciences 60(1):165–175

Krenzelok E P, Jacobsen T D, Aronis J 1997 American mistletoe exposures. American Journal of Emergency Medicine 15:516–520

*Motherwort* (Leonurus cardiaca) *(Lion's ear, Throw-wort)*

Traditional uses:   as a uterine stimulant for amenorrhoea and as a relaxant and cardiotonic, used for nervous tension, tachycardia.

Principal constituents:   alkaloids, bitters, glycosides, tannins, volatile oil, flavonoids, terpenoids, leonurine and stachydrine, ursolic acid.

Evidence:   There is some clinical evidence of its antibacterial and antioxidant properties.

Safety:   Side-effects from large oral doses include diarrhoea, stomach irritation and uterine bleeding; leaves can cause contact dermatitis and the oil can cause photosensitivity. Allergic reactions are possible in sensitive individuals. Cardiac glycoside toxicity is possible if used concomitantly with some herbs. There is a major risk of interaction with central nervous system depressants, which can potentiate the sedative and tranquillizing effects of these drugs, including antihistamines. Theoretically motherwort can trigger uterine bleeding, avoid in pregnancy and perimenopausal menorrhagia.

Bibliography

Soberón J R, Sgariglia M A, Sampietro D A et al 2007 Antibacterial activity of plant extracts from northwestern Argentina. Journal of Applied Microbiology 102(6):1450–1461

## Nettle (Urtica urens; Urtica dioica) *(also known as Great stinging nettle, Urtica)*

Traditional uses:  as a nutritive, haemostatic, astringent and circulatory stimulant for wound healing, for skin diseases, uterine haemorrhage and joint pains. It is particularly used for urinary problems, especially those associated with benign prostatic hyperplasia, including nocturia, frequency of micturition, dysuria, urinary retention and irritable bladder.

Principal constituents:  rich in vitamin C, K and minerals, particularly iron, flavonoids, lignans and amines.

Evidence:  Research on the use of nettle for benign prostatic hyperplasia is inconclusive but there is some evidence that it may be useful for osteoarthritis.

Safety:  Caution regarding concurrent medication, herbs and supplements with similar therapeutic actions. High vitamin K content may interfere with anticoagulant therapy. Side-effects of ingestion include gastrointestinal complaints, sweating and allergic skin reactions; localized rash, itching and stinging can arise from dermal application.

Bibliography

Alford L 2007 The use of nettle stings for pain. Alternative Therapies in Health and Medicine 13(6):58
Chrubasik J E, Roufogalis B D, Wagner H et al 2007 A comprehensive review on the stinging nettle effect and efficacy profiles. Part II: Urticae radix. Phytomedicine 14(7–8):568–579

Fagelman E, Lowe F C 2002 Herbal medications in the treatment of benign prostatic hyperplasia (BPH). Urologic Clinics in North America 29(1):23–29, vii

Gülçin I, Küfrevioglu O I, Oktay M et al 2004 Antioxidant, antimicrobial, antiulcer and analgesic activities of nettle (Urtica dioica L.). Journal of Ethnopharmacology 90(2–3):205–215

Lopatkin N, Sivkov A, Walther C 2005 Long-term efficacy and safety of a combination of sabal and urtica extract for lower urinary tract symptoms – a placebo-controlled, double-blind, multicenter trial. World Journal of Urology 23(2):139–146

Sahin M, Yilmaz H, Gursoy A 2007 Gynaecomastia in a man and hyperoestrogenism in a woman due to ingestion of nettle (Urtica dioica). New Zealand Medical Journal 120(1265), U2803

Testai L, Chericoni S, Calderone V 2002 Cardiovascular effects of Urtica dioica L. (Urticaceae) roots extracts: in vitro and in vivo pharmacological studies. Journal of Ethnopharmacology, 81(1):105–109

## Passion flower (Passiflora incarnata) *(also known as Passion vine, Passiflora, Passionblume, Apricot vine)*

Traditional uses: as a relaxant and antispasmodic, peripheral vasodilator and sedative, used for restlessness, irritability and insomnia, visceral tension and spasm.

Principal constituents: alkaloids, flavonoids, sterols and coumarins.

Evidence: There is some evidence which suggests passion flower is effective in cases of anxiety and anxiety-triggered disorders, as well as possibly for withdrawal from opiates.

Safety: Side-effects include dizziness, confusion, sedation and ataxia; vasculitis and altered consciousness have also been reported with commercial products derived mainly from passionflower fruit.

Avoid concomitant use with central nervous system depressants and with herbs that have sedative properties such as calamus, California poppy, catnip, hops, Jamaican dogwood, kava kava, St. John's wort, skullcap, valerian, yerba mate and others.

### Bibliography

Akhondzadeh S, Kashani L, Mobaseri M 2001 Passionflower in the treatment of opiates withdrawal: a double-blind randomized controlled trial. Journal of Clinical Pharmacy and Therapeutics 26(5):369–373

de Castro P C, Hoshino A, da Silva J C et al 2007 Possible anxiolytic effect of two extracts of Passiflora quadrangularis L. in experimental models. Phytotherapy Research 21(5):481–484

Dhawan K, Dhawan S, Sharma A 2004 Passiflora: a review update. Journal of Ethnopharmacology 94(1):1–23

Dhawan K, Kumar S, Sharma A 2003 Antiasthmatic activity of the methanol extract of leaves of Passiflora incarnata. Phytotherapy Research 17(7):821–822

Dhawan K, Sharma A 2002 Antitussive activity of the methanol extract of Passiflora incarnata leaves. Fitoterapia 73(5):397–399

Ernst E 2006 Herbal remedies for anxiety – a systematic review of controlled clinical trials. Phytomedicine 13(3):205–208

Miyasaka L S, Atallah A N, Soares B G 2007 Passiflora for anxiety disorder. Cochrane Database of Systematic Reviews(1):CD004518

## *Plantain* (Plantago major) *(also known as Common or Great plantain)*

Traditional uses:   Plantain has been used for cystitis with haematuria, bronchitis, colds and for irritated or bleeding hemorrhoids. It is also used as an antiseptic, antiinflammatory and antibacterial. Topically, great plantain is used for skin conditions and eye irritation or discomfort.

Principal constituents:   Low levels of tannins and relatively high concentrations of vitamin K, beta-carotene and calcium, as well as acids, amino acids, carbohydrates and iridoids.

Evidence:   Studies indicate antiinflammatory, antibacterial and antifungal properties. *In vitro* haematopoietic activity has also been demonstrated.

Safety:   Caution regarding concurrent medication, herbs and supplements with similar actions, particularly herbs which interfere with clotting mechanisms such as alfalfa, parsley and nettle. May interfere with warfarin absorption; avoid concomitant use. Not to be confused with Black Psyllium, Blond Psyllium, Buckhorn Plantain and Water Plantain.

Bibliography

Chiang L C, Chiang W, Chang M Y et al 2002 Antiviral activity of Plantago major extracts and related compounds in vitro. Antiviral Research 55(1):53–62

Holetz F B, Pessini G L, Sanches N R et al 2002 Screening of some plants used in the Brazilian folk medicine for the treatment of infectious diseases. Memórias do Instituto Oswaldo Cruz 97:1027–1031

Velasco-Lezama R, Tapia-Aguilar R, Román-Ramos R et al 2006 Effect of Plantago major on cell proliferation in vitro. Journal of Ethnopharmacology 103(1)

*Poke root* (Phytolacca americana) *(also known as Pokeweed, Cancer root, Red plant)*

Traditional uses:   as an emetic, anti-rheumatic anti-catarrhal, used for autoimmune, inflammatory and respiratory conditions such as tonsillitis, laryngitis. It is also used for mastitis, mumps, skin infections (scabies, tinea, sycosis, ringworm, acne), skin cancer, dysmenorrhoea and syphilis.

Constituents:   triterpenoid saponins, alkaloids, resins, tannins.

Evidence: There is some ongoing American research into the possibility that poke root may be useful for influenza and poliomyelitis, although no publications could be found to confirm this.

Safety:   Poke root should not be taken orally as toxicity can occur and there are some old case reports in the literature of poisoning from drinking tea made from this plant, thought to be due to proteinaceous mitogens, which may affect the thymus gland and the saponin glycosides, including phytolaccatoxin and phytolaccagenin, which cause gastrointestinal irritation. Adverse effects from ingestion include nausea, vomiting, cramping, abdominal pain, diarrhoea, haematemesis, hypotension, tachycardia, dyspnoea, urinary incontinence, convulsions, transient blindness, respiratory failure and death. Topical application may induce serious haematological alterations, such as plasmacytosis, mitotic changes in peripheral blood cells, eosinophilia, thrombocytopenia, abnormal platelet morphology and other haematological abnormalities. Protective gloves should be used to handle the plant.

---

Bibliography

There are some old case reports of adverse effects but no recent clinical literature could be found.

*Prickly ash* (Zanthoxylum americanum, Zanthoxylum cavaherculis) *(also known as Northern prickly ash, Angelica tree)*

Traditional uses:   Traditionally used for cramps, intermittent claudication, Raynaud's syndrome, chronic rheumatic conditions, hypotension, pyrexia, inflammation, as a stimulant, to ease toothache and for cancer (as an ingredient in Hoxsey cure).

Constituents: alkaloids, coumarins, resin, acid, volatile oil and tannins.

Evidence: Has been shown to be antifungal and antibacterial.

Safety: Caution regarding concurrent mediation, herbs and supplements with similar therapeutic action in particular any other herbs with diuretic properties which may further potentiate action. May increase the risk of bleeding in patients with bleeding disorders or taking anticoagulants including aspirin and NSAIDs. Not to be confused with angelica (Dong quai).

### Bibliography

Bafi-Yeboa N F, Arnason J T, Baker J et al 2005 Antifungal constituents of northern prickly ash, Zanthoxylum americanum mill. Phytomedicine 12(5):370–377

Gibbons S, Leimkugel J, Oluwatuyi M et al 2003 Activity of Zanthoxylum clava-herculis extracts against multi-drug resistant methicillin-resistant Staphylococcus aureus (mdr-MRSA). Phytotherapy Research 17(3):274–275

Ju Y, Still C C, Sacalis J N 2001 Cytotoxic coumarins and lignans from extracts of the Northern prickly ash (Zanthoxylum americanum). Phytotherapy Research 15(5):441–443

Smith M L, Gregory P, Bafi-Yeboa N F et al 2004 Inhibition of DNA polymerization and antifungal specificity of furanocoumarins present in traditional medicines. Photochemistry and Photobiology 79(6):506–509

*Psyllium* (Plantago psyllium, Psyllium indica) *(also known as Brown psyllium, Fleawort, French or Spanish psyllium, Plantain)*

Traditional uses: for chronic constipation and for softening stools in those with haemorrhoids, anal fissures, anorectal surgery and during pregnancy. It is also used orally for diarrhoea, irritable bowel syndrome, reducing raised cholesterol and for treating cancer.

Principal constituents: mucilages.

Evidence: Clinical studies demonstrate an effect on stool bulking, its benefit in colorectal conditions and cholesterol-lowering activity.

Safety: It is essential to take adequate fluid intake, as psyllium may cause oesophageal irritation when the seeds are eaten; they release a pigment that deposits in renal tubules which can be nephrotoxic. The pigment has been removed from most commercial products. May interact with diabetic medication, lithium and digoxin. It is thought to be safe in medicinal doses, up to 20g/day for up to 6 months. Side-effects include flatulence, diarrhoea, constipation, nausea, headache, backache, rhinitis and cough. Repeated use may cause chest congestion, hypotension, loss of consciousness or anaphylaxis.

### Bibliography

Chan M Y, Heng C K 2008 Sequential effects of a high-fiber diet with psyllium husks on the expression levels of hepatic genes and plasma lipids. Nutrition 24(1):57–66

Cicero A F, Derosa G, Manca M et al 2007 Different effect of psyllium and guar dietary supplementation on blood pressure control in hypertensive overweight patients: a six-month, randomized clinical trial. Clinical and Experimental Hypertension 29(6):383–394

Emami M H, Sayedyahossein S, Aslani A 2008 Safety and efficacy of new glyceryl trinitrate suppository formula: first double blind placebo-controlled clinical trial. Diseases of the Colon and Rectum 51(7):1079–1083

Khossousi A, Binns C W, Dhaliwal S S et al 2008 The acute effects of psyllium on postprandial lipaemia and thermogenesis in overweight and obese men. British Journal of Nutrition 99(5):1068–1075

King D E, Mainous A G 3rd, Egan B M, Woolson R F et al 2008 Effect of psyllium fiber supplementation on C-reactive protein: the trial to reduce inflammatory markers (TRIM). Annals of Family Medicine 6(2):100–106

Theuwissen E, Mensink R P 2008 Water-soluble dietary fibers and cardiovascular disease. Physiology and Behavior 94(2):285–292

Uehleke B, Ortiz M, Stange R 2008 Cholesterol reduction using psyllium husks – do gastrointestinal adverse effects limit compliance? Results of a specific observational study. Phytomedicine 15(3):153–159

### Raspberry leaf (Rubus idaeus) (also known as Red raspberry leaf)

Traditional uses:    to facilitate effective uterine action during childbirth; it has traditionally been ingested by pregnant women for many decades. It can also be used for other reproductive conditions, including 'morning sickness', prevention of miscarriage, dysmenorrhoea and menorrhagia. Raspberry leaf has also been used to treat vitamin deficiency, gastrointestinal and other disorders and topically for mouth and throat inflammation and skin rashes. It has recently been postulated that it may have a role in preventing or treating obesity.

Principal constituents:    tannins, flavonoids, ellagic and phenolic acids, anthocyanidins, ascorbic acid, beta-carotene, glutathione and alpha-tocopherol.

Evidence:   Research on the effectiveness and safety of raspberry leaf in pregnancy is inconclusive, although many surveys of antenatal use of herbs in general identify that women use it frequently. Studies have indicated antioxidant effects and veterinary research suggests that raspberry leaf has antibacterial properties.

Safety:   The uterine-enhancing effects of raspberry leaf are accumulative and women who wish to drink the tea to facilitate easier childbirth should start at 30–32 weeks' gestation, increasing gradually from one, to a maximum of four cups daily (the tea is more effective than commercially produced tablets). It should not be taken before the third trimester without the advice of a qualified medical herbalist. Dose-dependent excessive Braxton Hicks contractions are possible – if these occur, women should be advised to reduce the dose or to discontinue it completely. Pregnant women should not take raspberry leaf if they have a uterine scar from a previous Caesarean section or other uterine surgery or if they are due to have an elective Caesarean section for a medical or obstetric reason; if there is a history of preterm labour in this or a previous pregnancy or precipitate labour; or if there has been any antepartum haemorrhage in late pregnancy. It should also be avoided in women with breech presentation, multiple pregnancy, suspected cephalopelvic disproportion, hypertension. It may interfere with iron absorption and should be avoided in anyone taking antidepressants. Caution should also be used in people with hormone sensitive conditions due to the oestrogenic effects.

### Bibliography

Gudej J, Tomczyk M 2004 Determination of flavonoids, tannins and ellagic acid in leaves from Rubus L. species. Archives of Pharmacological Research 27(11):1114–1119

Morimoto C, Satoh Y, Hara M et al 2005 Anti-obese action of raspberry ketone. Life Sciences 77(2):194–204

Parsons M, Simpson M, Ponton T 1999 Raspberry leaf and its effects on labour: safety and efficacy. Australian College of Midwives Incorporated Journal 12:20–25

Patel A V, Rojas-Vera J, Dacke C G 2004 Therapeutic constituents and actions of Rubus species. Current Medicinal Chemistry 11(11):1501–1512

Rojas-Vera J, Patel A V, Dacke C G 2002 Relaxant activity of raspberry (Rubus idaeus) leaf extract in guinea-pig ileum in vitro. Phytotherapy Research 16(7):665–668

Ryan T, Wilkinson J M, Cavanagh H M 2001 Antibacterial activity of raspberry cordial in vitro. Research in Veterinary Science 71(3):155–159

Simpson M, Parsons M, Greenwood J et al 2001 Raspberry leaf in pregnancy: its safety and efficacy in labor. Journal of Midwifery and Women's Health 46:51–59

Wang S Y, Lin H S 2000 Antioxidant activity in fruits and leaves of blackberry, raspberry and strawberry varies with cultivar and developmental stage. Journal of Agricultural and Food Chemistry 48:140–146

## Red clover (Trefolium pratense) *(also known as Beebread, Cow clover, Genistein, Isoflavone, Meadow or Wild clover)*

Traditional uses:    for perimenopausal symptoms, particularly hot flushes and mastalgia and for premenstrual syndrome, but it is also used for indigestion, hypercholesterolaemia, sexually transmitted diseases and some respiratory conditions.

Principal constituents:    coumarins, flavonoids, phenolic glycosides, cyanogenic glycosides.

Evidence:    Studies indicate antiinflammatory properties and a possible protective effect against atherosclerosis. Trials on red clover for perimenopausal symptoms have had variable results but recent research suggests that it is safe and may have some benefits in perimenopausal women, even when there is a family history of breast cancer, which was previously thought to be a contraindication to phytotherapeutic remedies, in the same way as hormone replacement therapy is contraindicated.

Safety:    Red clover is safe to take orally for up to 1 year. It should be avoided in pregnancy due to the oestrogenic effects. Side-effects include headache, nausea, vaginal spotting, skin rashes. It may increase the risk of endometrial hyperplasia but does not appear to increase risk of endometrial cancer. Avoid concomitant use with anticoagulant drugs and herbs such as clove, dong quai, garlic, ginger, ginkgo, Panax ginseng, horse chestnut, turmeric, as well as with herbs which have possible oestrogenic activity, e.g. alfalfa, black cohosh, chasteberry, flaxseed, hops, licorice, soy. There is a moderate possibility that red clover will interact with the contraceptive Pill and tamoxifen.

### Bibliography

Albertazzi P 2007 Non-estrogenic approaches for the treatment of climacteric symptoms. Climacteric 10(Suppl 2):115–120

Chedraui P, Hidalgo L, San Miguel G 2006 Red clover extract (MF11RCE) supplementation and postmenopausal vaginal and sexual health. International Journal of Gynaecology and Obstetrics 95(3):296–297

Cheema D, Coomarasamy A, El-Toukhy T 2007 Non-hormonal therapy of post-menopausal vasomotor symptoms: a structured evidence-based review. Archives of Gynecology and Obstetrics 276(5):463–469

Engelhardt P F, Riedl C R 2008 Effects of one-year treatment with isoflavone extract from red clover on prostate, liver function, sexual function and quality of life in men with elevated PSA levels and negative prostate biopsy findings. Urology 71(2):185–190

Occhiuto F, Pasquale R D, Guglielmo G 2007 Effects of phytoestrogenic isoflavones from red clover (Trifolium pratense L.) on experimental osteoporosis. Phytotherapy Research 21(2):130–134

Tempfer C B, Bentz E K, Leodolter S 2007 Phytoestrogens in clinical practice: a review of the literature. Fertility and Sterility 87(6):1243–1249

Umland E M 2008 Treatment strategies for reducing the burden of menopause-associated vasomotor symptoms. Journal of Managed Care Pharmacy 14(Suppl): 14–19

## Rue (Ruta graveolens) *(also known as German rue, Herb of grace)*

Traditional uses:   for menstrual disorders, as a uterine stimulant and abortifacient, for loss of appetite and dyspepsia, for arteriosclerosis, heart palpitations and nervousness, for infectious diseases with pyrexia, respiratory conditions and intestinal worm infestations. Rue is also used as an antispasmodic, diuretic, antibacterial and antifungal and as a contraceptive agent.

Principal constituents:   volatile oil, flavonoids, furanocoumarins, alkaloids and tannins.

Evidence:   Rue has been shown to be antimicrobial and antibacterial. Animal studies suggest a possible anti-arrhythmic effect and *in vitro* investigations have identified a potential use of rue as a new male contraceptive agent. There is also promising evidence of anti-tumour effects.

Safety:   May increase the risk of bleeding in patients with bleeding disorders or taking anticoagulants including aspirin and non-steroidal antiinflammatories. Contraindicated in pregnancy. Side-effects include depression, insomnia and tiredness, dizziness, spasms, gastrointestinal irritation, convulsions, severe renal and hepatic damage and death. Doses should be kept below 120g of the leaf to avoid severe consequences.

Contact dermatitis and phototoxic reactions may occur with topical exposure to the fresh plant and rue-containing products followed by exposure to sunlight.

### Bibliography

Al-Heali F M, Rahemo Z 2006 The combined effect of two aqueous extracts on the growth of Trichomonas vaginalis, in vitro. Turkish Society for Parasitology 30(4):272–274

Eickhorst K, DeLeo V, Csaposs J 2007 Rue the herb: Ruta graveolens – associated phytophototoxicity. Dermatitis 18(1):52–55

Harat Z N, Sadeghi M R, Sadeghipour H R et al 2008 Immobilization effect of Ruta graveolens L. on human sperm: a new hope for male contraception. Journal of Ethnopharmacology 115(1):36–41

Nogueira J C, Diniz Mde F, Lima E O 2008 In vitro antimicrobial activity of plants in Acute Otitis Externa. Revista brasileira de otorrinolaringologia (English ed.) 74(1):118–124

Preethi K C, Kuttan G, Kuttan R 2006 Anti-tumour activity of Ruta graveolens extract. Asian Pacific Journal of Cancer Prevention 7(3):439–443

Réthy B, Zupkó I, Minorics R et al 2007 Investigation of cytotoxic activity on human cancer cell lines of arborinine and furanoacridones isolated from Ruta graveolens. Planta Medica 73(1):41–48

*Sage* (Salvia officinale, Salvia lavandulaefolia) *(also known as Common or True sage, Dalmatian or Spanish sage, Garden or Meadow sage)*

Traditional uses:    for loss of appetite, gastritis, diarrhoea, flatulence and excessive salivation, for excessive perspiration and hot flushes, especially during the menopause, for dysmenorrhoea and galactorrhoea, for depression, poor memory and in Alzheimer's disease. It is also claimed to be helpful as an inhalation for respiratory conditions including, colds, influenza and asthma.

Principal constituents:    volatile oils, oestrogenic substances, triterpenoid saponins, flavonoids, tannins, resin, camphor and thujone.

Evidence:    There is some evidence that sage can be effective in memory enhancement in people with Alzheimer's disease. It has also been shown to be effective against various viruses including herpes simplex.

Safety:    Sage is thought to be safe when used in cooking and for up to four months as a medicinal product. It is contraindicated during menstruation, in the preconception period, during pregnancy and when breastfeeding. Contraindicated in epileptics – some species of sage contain thujone which is neurotoxic. The camphor content may be hepatotoxic, neurotoxic and abortifacient. Should not be taken concomitantly with anti-diabetic medication, sedatives or drugs which depress the central nervous system. Do not confuse with clary sage, German sarsaparilla, Greek sage or wood sage.

Bibliography

Büyükbalci A, El S N 2008 Determination of in vitro antidiabetic effects, antioxidant activities and phenol contents of some herbal teas. Plant Foods and Human Nutrition 63(1):27–33

Hellum B H, Nilsen O G 2007 The in vitro inhibitory potential of trade herbal products on human CYP2D6-mediated metabolism and the influence of ethanol. Basic Clinical Pharmacology and Toxicology 101(5):350–358

Roberts A T, Martin C K, Liu Z 2007 The safety and efficacy of a dietary herbal supplement and gallic acid for weight loss. Journal of Medicinal Food 10(1): 184–188

Scholey A B, Tildesley N T, Ballard C G 2008 An extract of Salvia (sage) with anticholinesterase properties improves memory and attention in healthy older volunteers. Psychopharmacology (Berl) 198(1):127–139

*Saw palmetto* (Serenoa serrulata) *(also known as American dwarf palm tree, Cabbage palm)*

Traditional uses:  as a diuretic and urinary antiseptic; specifically used for benign prostatic hyperplasia, as well as chronic or subacute cystitis, testicular atrophy and sex hormone disorders.

Principal constituents: volatile oils, steroidal saponins, resins, tannins, fixed oil, alkaloid.

Evidence:  *In vitro* animal and clinical trials indicate the prevention of testosterone converting to dihydrotestosterone as inhibitory effects on androgen receptors and antiinflammatory properties. It reduces symptoms of benign prostate hypertrophy without reducing the size of the prostate and has been shown to be safe in studies lasting up to a year. Anticoagulant.

Safety: Caution regarding concurrent medication, herbs and supplements with similar therapeutic effect in particular those with diuretic properties which may potentiate the effects. May increase the risk of haemorrhage in patients with bleeding disorders or taking anticoagulants including aspirin and non-steroidal antiinflammatories. May cause erectile dysfunction, ejaculatory disturbance or altered libido.

Bibliography

Avins A L, Bent S 2006 Saw palmetto and lower urinary tract symptoms: what is the latest evidence? Current Urology Reports 7(4):260–265

Bonnar-Pizzorno R M, Littman A J, Kestin M et al 2006 Saw palmetto supplement use and prostate cancer risk. Nutrition Cancer 55(1):21–27

McVary K T 2006 Saw palmetto for benign prostatic hyperplasia. Current Urology Reports 7(4):251

Shi R, Xie Q, Gang X 2008 Effect of saw palmetto soft gel capsule on lower urinary tract symptoms associated with benign prostatic hyperplasia: a randomized trial in Shanghai, China. Journal of Urology 179(2):610–615

Ulbricht C, Basch E, Bent S et al 2006 Evidence-based systematic review of saw palmetto by the Natural Standard Research Collaboration. Journal of Society Integrative Oncology 4(4):170–186

Webber R 2006 Benign prostatic hyperplasia. Clinical Evidence 15:1213–1226

## *Skullcap* (Scutellaria laterifolia)

Traditional uses:   nervous system relaxant and restorative, sedative, antispasmodic; used for neurological and neuro-motor conditions including epilepsy, nervous exhaustion and debility.

Principal constituents:   flavonoids, iridoids, tannins, volatile oil.

Evidence:   *In vitro* animal studies and clinical trials indicate antiinflammatory, CNS depressant, antiviral properties.

Safety:   Caution regarding concurrent medication, herbs and supplements with similar therapeutic action including diuretic herbs which may potentiate the effects. Caution with concurrent sedation and analgesics containing codeine.

Bibliography

Awad R, Arnason J T, Trudeau V 2003 Phytochemical and biological analysis of skullcap (Scutellaria lateriflora L.): a medicinal plant with anxiolytic properties. Phytomedicine 10(8):640–649

Dedhia R C, McVary K T 2008 Phytotherapy for lower urinary tract symptoms secondary to benign prostatic hyperplasia. Journal of Urology 179(6):2119–2125

Shi R, Xie Q, Gang X et al 2008 Effect of saw palmetto soft gel capsule on lower urinary tract symptoms associated with benign prostatic hyperplasia: a randomized trial in Shanghai, China. Journal of Urology 179(2):610–615

Wojcikowski K, Stevenson L, Leach D et al 2007 Antioxidant capacity of 55 medicinal herbs traditionally used to treat the urinary system: a comparison using a sequential three-solvent extraction process. Journal of Alternative Complementary Medicine 13(1):103–109

## Slippery elm (Ulmus fulva) *(also known as Red elm)*

Traditional uses: as a soothing agent for irritated mucosa including sore throats and coughs, for sickness in pregnancy, as a nutritional supplement during convalescence and topically for boils and abscesses.

Principal constituents: tannins, mucilages, oleoresins.

Evidence: There is some suggestion that slippery elm may have antioxidant effects.

Safety: Slippery elm is a component of essiac, please refer to other listing.

### Bibliography

Langmead L, Dawson C, Hawkins C 2002 Antioxidant effects of herbal therapies used by patients with inflammatory bowel disease: an in vitro study. Alimentary Pharmacology and Therapeutics 16(2):197–205

## St John's wort (Hypericum perforatum)

Traditional uses: as an antidepressant, gentle and calming, nervous tonic and restorative used for anxiety states, tension and irritability, external wound application.

Principal constituents: glycosides, flavonoids, tannins, resin and volatile oil, hypericin.

Evidence: *In vitro* animal studies and clinical trials indicate antidepressant effects for people with mild to moderate, but not severe, depression. It has also been shown to be antimicrobial in high concentrations (*Staphylococcus aureus, Streptococcus pyogenes*) and has antiinflammatory and wound healing properties. There is some suggestion that it may relieve symptoms of the perimenopausal period but there is insufficient evidence to date to determine its effects in premenstrual syndrome.

Safety: Should not be used concomitantly with SSRIs, tricyclic anti-depressants, antipsychotics, benzodiazepines oral hypoglycaemic agents, angiotensin II receptor antagonists, proton pump inhibitors, antihistamines, warfarin, cardiac glycosides, anticonvulsants and the contraceptive Pill. Avoid during the preconception period, pregnancy and lactation. Side-effects include insomnia and fatigue, vivid dreams, anxiety, agitation and irritability, gastrointestinal disorders, dizziness and headache, skin rashes, paraesthesia and hypoglycaemia. In depressed patients it can induce hypomania or mania in those with bipolar disorder. Photosensitivity is a significant side-effect from topical administration and from long-term oral use, notably in fair-skinned people. There have also been a few isolated cases of St John's wort triggering serotonin syndrome involving extreme anxiety, confusion, nausea, hypertension and tachycardia. As with SSRIs, male sexual dysfunction may occur. St John's wort should not be discontinued abruptly; doses should be decreased gradually.

### Bibliography

Dugoua J J, Mills E, Perri D et al 2006 Safety and efficacy of St. John's wort (Hypericum) during pregnancy and lactation. Canadian Journal of Clinical Pharmacology, 13(3):e268–e276

Gurley B J, Swain A, Hubbard M A et al 2008 Clinical assessment of CYP2D6-mediated herb-drug interactions in humans: effects of milk thistle, black cohosh, goldenseal, kava kava, St. John's wort and Echinacea. Molecular Nutrition and Food Research 52(7):755–763

Hellum B H, Nilsen O G 2007 The in vitro inhibitory potential of trade herbal products on human CYP2D6-mediated metabolism and the influence of ethanol. Basic and Clinical Pharmacology and Toxicology 101(5):350–358

Izzo A A, Di Carlo G, Borrelli F et al 2005 Cardiovascular pharmacotherapy and herbal medicines: the risk of drug interaction. International Journal of Cardiology 98(1):1–14

Mannucci C, Pieratti A, Firenzuoli F 2007 Serotonin mediates beneficial effects of Hypericum perforatum on nicotine withdrawal signs. Phytomedicine 14(10): 645–651

Papakostas G I, Crawford C M, Scalia M J et al 2007 Timing of clinical improvement and symptom resolution in the treatment of major depressive disorder. A replication of findings with the use of a double-blind, placebo-controlled trial of Hypericum perforatum versus fluoxetine. Neuropsychobiology 56(2–3):132–137

Saeed S A, Bloch R M, Antonacci D J 2007 Herbal and dietary supplements for treatment of anxiety disorders. American Family Physician 76(4):549–556

Sarino L V, Dang K H, Dianat N 2007 Drug interaction between oral contraceptives and St. John's wort: appropriateness of advice received from community pharmacists and health food store clerks. Journal of the American Pharmaceutic Association 47(1):42–47

Shalansky S, Lynd L, Richardson K et al 2007 Risk of warfarin-related bleeding events and supratherapeutic international normalized ratios associated with complementary and alternative medicine: a longitudinal analysis. Pharmacotherapy 27(9):1237–1247

Uzbay T I 2008 Hypericum perforatum and substance dependence: a review. Phytotherapy Research 22(5):578–582

## Turmeric (Curcuma longa) *(Indian saffron)*

Traditional uses:  as an antiinflammatory agent for gastrointestinal conditions, hepatic disorders, arthritis, irritable bowel syndrome and for local application for cancerous lesions and cancer prevention.

Principal constituents:  curcuminoid compounds.

Evidence:  Studies indicate antiinflammatory, hypotensive, anticoagulant, hypocholesterolaemic and cancer preventative properties.

Safety:  May increase the risk of bleeding in people with bleeding disorders or taking anticoagulants including aspirin and non-steroidal antiinflammatories and may interfere with tricyclic antidepressants, antipsychotics, benzodiazepines, oral hypoglycaemic agents, angiotensin II receptor antagonists, proton pump inhibitors, antihistamines. May compromise the immune system and may increase the risk of renal calculi.

### Bibliography

Baum L, Lam C W, Cheung S K et al 2008 Six-month randomized, placebo-controlled, double-blind, pilot clinical trial of curcumin in patients with Alzheimer disease. Journal of Clinical Psychopharmacology 28(1):110–113

Jantan I, Raweh S M, Sirat H M 2008 Inhibitory effect of compounds from Zingiberaceae species on human platelet aggregation. Phytomedicine 15(4): 306–309

Menon V P, Sudheer A R 2007 Antioxidant and anti-inflammatory properties of curcumin. Advances Experimental Medicine Biology 595:105–125

Miriyala S, Panchatcharam M, Rengarajulu P 2007 Cardioprotective effects of curcumin. Advances in Experimental Medicine and Biology 595:359–377

Rao C V 2007 Regulation of COX and LOX by curcumin. Advances in Experimental Medicine and Biology 595:213–226

Tang M, Larson-Meyer D E, Liebman M 2008 Effect of cinnamon and turmeric on urinary oxalate excretion, plasma lipids and plasma glucose in healthy subjects. American Journal of Clinical Nutrition 87(5):1262–1267

Venkatesan N, Punithavathi D, Babu M 2007 Protection from acute and chronic lung diseases by curcumin. Advances in Experimental Medicine and Biology 595:379–405

*Valerian* (Valeriana officinalis) *(also known as All-heal, Garden heliotrope)*

Traditional uses:   as a tranquillizer and sedative for insomnia, anxiety states, mood disorders and other stress- and anxiety-related conditions such as headache, hysteria and muscle tension.

Principal constituents:   volatile oils, alkaloids, iridoids, resins, valepotriates.

Evidence:   suggests that valerian is effective for sleep-related disorders but its value for anxiety conditions has not been adequately demonstrated. Trials have shown it to be sedative-hypnotic, anxiolytic, antidepressant, anticonvulsant, antispasmodic and possibly hypotensive.

Safety:   Side-effects include headache, excitability, vivid dreams, cardiac disturbances, insomnia, gastrointestinal disorders and morning drowsiness. People who take valerian at night should be warned to take care when driving or operating machinery the following morning. Valerian should be discontinued gradually. Several cases of hepatotoxicity have been reported, although these were in people who ingested valerian in combination with other herbal sedatives; however, it is probably wise to refrain from taking valerian in the presence of liver disease.

### Bibliography

Awad R, Levac D, Cybulska P 2007 Effects of traditionally used anxiolytic botanicals on enzymes of the gamma-aminobutyric acid (GABA) system. Canadian Journal of Physiology Pharmacology 85(9):933–942

Babic D 2007 Herbal medicine in the treatment of mental disorders. Psychiatric Danube 19(3):241–244

Gooneratne N S 2008 Complementary and alternative medicine for sleep disturbances in older adults. Clinical Geriatric Medicine 24(1):121–138, viii

Hattesohl M, Feistel B, Sievers H 2008 Extracts of Valeriana officinalis L. s.l. show anxiolytic and antidepressant effects but neither sedative nor myorelaxant properties. Phytomedicine 15(1–2):2–15

Hellum B H, Nilsen O G 2007 The in vitro inhibitory potential of trade herbal products on human CYP2D6-mediated metabolism and the influence of ethanol. Basic and Clinical Pharmacology and Toxicology 101(5):350–358

Meolie A L, Rosen C, Kristo D; Clinical Practice Review Committee; American Academy of Sleep Medicine 2005 Oral nonprescription treatment for insomnia: an evaluation of products with limited evidence. Journal of Clinical Sleep Medicine 1(2):173–187

Taibi D M, Landis C A, Petry H et al 2007 A systematic review of valerian as a sleep aid: safe but not effective. Sleep Medicine Reviews 11(3):209–230

*Wild lettuce* (Lactuca virosa) *(also known as Green endive)*

Traditional uses:   as a mild peripheral dilator and antiinflammatory agent, principally for respiratory tract conditions such as mucus membrane inflammation, bronchitis and whooping cough, as well as urinary problems, menstrual and childbirth cramps and for some sexual disorders.

Principal constituents:   triterpenes, alkaloid, coumarins, terpenoids, flavonoids.

Evidence:   There is some suggestion that wild lettuce has sedative properties.

Safety:   Side-effects include sweating, increased respiration, tachycardia, dilated pupils, tinnitus, visual disorders, headaches, respiratory depression, coma and death. Applied topically, dermatitis can occur and allergic reaction to wild lettuce has developed in some people sensitive to other plants such as marigolds, daisies and chrysanthemums. There is considerable risk of interaction with central nervous system depressants and there is concern that it may contain hyoscyamine which is contraindicated in conditions involving urinary retention, therefore it should not be taken by men with prostate enlargement.

Bibliography

Meolie A L, Rosen C, Kristo D; Clinical Practice Review Committee; American Academy of Sleep Medicine 2005 Oral nonprescription treatment for insomnia: an evaluation of products with limited evidence. Journal of Clinical Sleep Medicine 1(2):173–187

Paulsen E, Andersen K E, Hausen B M 2001 Sensitization and cross-reaction patterns in Danish Compositae-allergic patients. Contact Dermatitis 45(4):197–204.

*Wild yam* (Dioscorea villosa) *(also known as China root, Mexican yam, Shan Yao)*

Traditional uses:   as a 'natural alternative' for hormone replacement therapy, for postmenopausal vaginal dryness, hot flushes, premenstrual syndrome and dysmenorrhoea, osteoporosis, increasing energy and libido in men and women and for breast enlargement.

Principal constituents:   diosgenin, now used as a precursor for commercial preparation of human steroidal drugs, steroidal saponins, alkaloids, tannins and starch.

Evidence:    *In vitro* animal and clinical studies indicate hypoglycaemic, hypocholesterolaemic and uterine stimulation properties.

Safety: Nausea and vomiting has been reported in those taking prolonged courses of wild yam. Should not be taken in pregnancy or by those with hormone-sensitive conditions. The diosgenin in wild yam is often promoted as a natural precursor to dehydroepiandrosterone (DHEA) and some wild yam commercial products are labelled 'natural DHEA.' However, although diosgenin can be converted to DHEA *in vitro*, this process is not thought to occur in the human body, therefore wild yam extract will not increase DHEA levels. Wild yam should not be confused with bitter yam.

### Bibliography

Carroll D G 2006 Nonhormonal therapies for hot flashes in menopause. American Family Physician 73(3):457–464

Komesaroff P A, Black C V, Cable V et al 2001 Effects of wild yam extract on menopausal symptoms, lipids and sex hormones in healthy menopausal women. Climacteric 4(2):144–150

Laveaga G S 2005 Uncommon trajectories: steroid hormones, Mexican peasants and the search for a wild yam. Studies in History and Philosophy of Biological and Biomedical Sciences 36(4):743–760

Russell L, Hicks G S, Low A K 2002 Phytoestrogens: a viable option? American Journal of Medical Science 324(4):185–188

*Willow bark* (Salix alba) *(also known as Black/White/Purple willow)*

Traditional uses:    as an antiinflammatory, analgesic, astringent and local antiseptic. It has been used for arthritis, rheumatism, headache, gout, neuralgia and as an antipyretic.

Principal constituents:    salicylates, tannins, glycosides, flavonoids.

Evidence:    There is some evidence of its analgesic effects in people with backache, but its value in arthritic disorders has not been confirmed.

Safety:    Should not be used in patients with haemorrhagic disorders, taking anticoagulants, those with gastric or duodenal ulcers, during pregnancy and lactation or in children under 12 years of age. Dermatitis, skin rashes and allergic reactions have been reported; those allergic to aspirin should not take willow bark. Salicylates can inhibit prostaglandins, which reduce renal blood flow and the salicin content can cause renal papillary necrosis. It should not be taken concomitantly with other herbs which have anticoagulant effects, including clove, garlic, ginger, ginkgo, ginseng, meadowsweet and red clover, nor with those containing salicylates, such as black haw and poplar. It should be used with caution in people with asthma, diabetes, gout and kidney or liver disease.

### Bibliography

Biegert C, Wagner I, Lüdtke R 2004 Efficacy and safety of willow bark extract in the treatment of osteoarthritis and rheumatoid arthritis: results of 2 randomized double-blind controlled trials. Journal of Rheumatology 31(11):2121–2130

Chrubasik S, Künzel O, Model A et al 2001 Treatment of low back pain with a herbal or synthetic anti-rheumatic: a randomized controlled study. Willow bark extract for low back pain. Rheumatology (Oxford) 40(12):1388–1393

Setty A R, Sigal L H 2005 Herbal medications commonly used in the practice of rheumatology: mechanisms of action, efficacy and side-effects. Seminars Arthritis Rheumatology 34(6):773–784

Shalansky S, Lynd L, Richardson K et al 2007 Risk of warfarin-related bleeding events and supratherapeutic international normalized ratios associated with complementary and alternative medicine: a longitudinal analysis. Pharmacotherapy 27(9):1237–1247

*Witch hazel* (Hamamelis virginiana) *(also known as Hamamelis, Tobacco wood, Spotted elder)*

Traditional uses:   for diarrhoea, colitis, haematemesis or haemoptysis, tuberculosis, colds, fevers, tumors and cancer. Topically, witch hazel is used for skin itching, inflammation and injury, mucous membrane inflammation, varicose veins, haemorrhoids, bruises, insect bites, minor burns and other skin irritations.

Principal constituents:   mixed tannins, bitters, volatile oil, flavonoids, saponins.

Evidence:   Studies indicate astringent and haemostatic properties and its value in treating haemorrhoids and eczema.

Safety:   Taken orally, gastrointestinal disturbances, kidney damage and hepatic necrosis may occur and prolonged ingestion of tannin-containing herbs can lead to certain cancers. However, topical administration is thought to be safe, although dermatitis can develop in susceptible people.

Bibliography

East C E, Begg L, Henshall N E 2007 Local cooling for relieving pain from perineal trauma sustained during childbirth. Cochrane Database of Systematic Reviews(4), CD006304

Iauk L, Lo Bue A M, Milazzo I et al 2003 Antibacterial activity of medicinal plant extracts against periodontopathic bacteria. Phytotherapy Research 17(6):599–604

Paulsen E, Chistensen L P, Andersen K E 2008 Cosmetics and herbal remedies with Compositae plant extracts – are they tolerated by Compositae-allergic patients? Contact Dermatitis 58(1):15–23

Touriño S, Lizárraga D, Carreras A et al 2008 Highly galloylated tannin fractions from witch hazel (Hamamelis virginiana) bark: electron transfer capacity, in vitro antioxidant activity and effects on skin-related cells. Chemical Research in Toxicology 21(3):696–704

Wolff H H, Kieser M 2007 Hamamelis in children with skin disorders and skin injuries: results of an observational study. European Journal of Pediatrics 166(9):943–948

## Yerba maté (Ilex paraguariensis) *(also known as Jesuits Brazil tree, Paraguay tree, Maté)*

Traditional uses:   nervous headaches due to fatigue, appetite reduction, day time stimulant to induce sleep at night, mild analgesia.

Principal constituents:   alkaloids including caffeine, tannins and volatile oils.

Evidence:   Animal and clinical studies indicate hypotensive, central nervous system stimulant and antiviral activity. The effects of xanthine constituents, notably caffeine, are well documented including cardiac stimulation, coronary dilation, smooth muscle relaxation and diuresis.

Safety:   Caution regarding concurrent medication, herbs and supplements with similar therapeutic actions. Caution with concurrent ingestion of caffeine; commercial preparations may contain high concentrations of caffeine.

Bibliography

Andrews K W, Schweitzer A, Zhao C et al 2007 The caffeine contents of dietary supplements commonly purchased in the US: analysis of 53 products with caffeine-containing ingredients. Analytical and Bioanalytical Chemistry 389(1):231–239

Heck C I, de Mejia E G 2007 Yerba Mate Tea (Ilex paraguariensis): a comprehensive review on chemistry, health implications and technological considerations. Journal of Food Science 2(9):R138–R151

Menini T, Heck C, Schulze J et al 2007 Protective action of Ilex paraguariensis extract against free radical inactivation of paraoxonase-1 in high-density lipoprotein. Planta Medica 73(11):1141–1147

Müller V, Chávez J H, Reginatto F H et al 2007 Evaluation of antiviral activity of South American plant extracts against herpes simplex virus type 1 and rabies virus. Phytotherapy Research 21(10):970–974

Pittler M H, Schmidt K, Ernst E 2005 Adverse events of herbal food supplements for body weight reduction: systematic review. Obesity Review 6(2):93–111

# Homeopathy

## Description

Homeopathy is a system of vibrational or energy medicine based on the concept of 'like curing like' developed and refined by Samuel Hahnemann (1755–1843), the term derived from the Greek *homoios* (same) and *pathos* (illness). Unicist or classical homeopathy uses only single remedies in a single prescription, whereas complex homeopathy uses remedies in combination. In clinical homeopathy, remedies are prescribed according to individual symptoms rather than the totality of symptoms. In isopathy, the presenting symptom picture is ignored, the remedy given being the substance thought to have caused the symptoms in the first place. According to Hering's Law, symptoms are said to resolve in the reverse order of their onset, from above downwards and from inside outwards.

Remedies are prepared by being serially diluted and succussed (vigorously shaken) which is thought to transmit the energy of the substance into the water in which it has been diluted. The strength (dosage) is denoted by the letters X, C, M and LM indicating the level of dilution to the power of 10, 100, 1000, etc. and by numbers 6, 30, 100, 200, etc. which indicate the number of times the substance has been diluted and succussed. The higher the number and letter, the more dilute the remedy, in chemical (pharmacological) terms, yet the more potent it becomes in homeopathic terms. Treatment aims to use the minimal dose possible required to produce a therapeutic effect. Remedies are then administered as pilules, granules, crystals, individual powders, liquids, mother tinctures, ointments, creams, lotions and liniments. The unique method of testing the efficacy of a homeopathic remedy is by administrating the remedy to a number of healthy subjects and noting their reactions to the remedy, which then gives the full symptom picture which can be treated by the homeopathic dilution of the substance.

Constitutional remedies:    prescribed according to the principle that people with certain common, easily identifiable constitutional patterns have a higher propensity for certain chronic illnesses and are prescribed at the onset of an illness to enhance the person's resistance. As far as is possible, the remedy picture is matched to the patient's constitutional (or characteristic) pattern as well as the presenting symptoms. Polychrest remedies are based on the individual's constitutional type but also have a wide clinical application affecting nearly all of the body's tissues and are indicated for both acute and chronic conditions.

A concept which is not accepted by all homeopaths but which is influential in classical homeopathy is that of miasmas. Hahnemann identified three miasmas, syphilis (breakdown or disorganization), sycosis (excessive or over reaction) and psora (deficiency or under reaction) which he considered to be the acquired or inherited cause of all chronic diseases. Miasmas act either singly or in combination, leading to a predisposition to certain chronic illnesses or conditions. Later miasmas included tubercular diathesis and cancerinic miasma.

Evidence:    There is some evidence to suggest that homeopathic remedies have a part to play in the treatment of some conditions, although many trials are not randomized controlled studies and are therefore not easily accepted by conventional medical professionals, the effects of homeopathy being attributed to the placebo effect. However, there is considerable evidence for the use of homeopathic remedies in veterinary medicine. In view of the number of individual remedies and the paucity of evidence on specific remedies, only those for which contemporary literature could be found have been included in the following section on Selected Homeopathic remedies.

Safety:    There are no contraindications or interactions with orthodox medication or treatment remedies, although therapeutic aggravation may occur which is not a side-effect but usually denotes that the correct remedy has been selected for the individual. As the remedies are chemically fragile, there are several substances which should be avoided while using homeopathic treatment, including mint products such as toothpaste, coffee, strongly aromatic substances including essential oils and heat liniments for muscular pain. Remedies should only be handled by the person for whom they are intended and should not be administered on a metal spoon. Homeopathy is safe for children and in pregnancy but dilutions further away from the original substance, e.g. 30C rather than 6C, may be wise. Remedies are lactose-based and should not be used by people with lactose intolerance. Homeopathy should not be used as a substitute for orthodox treatment for life-threatening situations. Care should be taken not to confuse the homeopathic preparation of a remedy with the herbal remedy of the same name which acts pharmacologically and can be extremely dangerous, given that some substances used in homeopathy are derived from potentially toxic substances, e.g. arsenic.

## Bibliography

Anick D 2007 The octave potencies convention: a mathematical model of dilution and succession. Homeopathy 96(3):202–208

Bell I, Baldwin C, Schwartz G 2002 Translating a nonlinear systems theory model for homeopathy into empirical tests. Alternative Therapies in Health and Medicine 8(3):58–66

Chaplin M 2007 The memory of water: an overview. Homeopathy 96(3):143–150

Cucherat M, Haugh M, Gooch M et al 2000 Evidence of clinical efficacy of homeopathy: a meta-analysis of clinical trials. European Journal of Clinical Pharmacology 56:27–33

Itamura R 2007 Effect of homeopathic treatment of 60 Japanese patients with chronic skin disease. Complementary Therapies in Medicine 15(2):115–120

Mohan G 2007 Efficacy of homeopathy in childhood asthmas. Homeopath-Links 20(2):104–107

Owen J, Green B 2004 Homeopathic treatment of headaches: a systematic review of the literature. Journal of Chiropractic Medicine 3:45–52

Pilkington K, Kirkwood G, Rampes H et al 2005 Homeopathy for depression: a systematic review of the research evidence. Homeopathy 94:153–163

Pilkington K, Kirkwood G, Rampes H 2006 Homeopathy for anxiety and anxiety disorders: a systematic review of the research. Homeopathy 95:151–162

Shang A, Huwiler-Muntener K, Nartey L 2005 Are the clinical effects of homeopathy placebo effects? Comparative study of placebo-controlled trials of homeopathy and allopathy. Lancet 366:726–732

Taylor M, Reilly D, Llewellyn-Jones R et al 2000 Randomised controlled trials of homeopathy versus placebo in perennial allergic rhinitis with over view of four trial series. British Medical Journal 321:471–476

Weingartner O 2007 The nature of the active ingredient in ultra-molecular dilutions. Homeopathy 96(3):220–226

### Resources

Faculty of Homeopathy and British Homeopathic Association: www.trusthomeopathy.org

Society of Homeopaths: www.homeopathy-soh.org

## Selected homeopathic remedies

### Aconite (Aconitum napellus)

Constitutional remedy reflecting characteristics of low self esteem, tendency to insensitivity and fear of crowds; prepared from the plant known as monk's hood or wolf's bane. Prescribed for severe shock or fright, palpitations, central chest pain with feelings of impending doom, acute onset of infections, sudden onset of severe headaches, general burning pains and numbness, upper respiratory tract infections in children.

Evidence:    May be of value in the treatment of otitis media.

Safety:    No specific safety information.

Bibliography

Friese K H, Kruse S, Lüdtke R 1997 The homoeopathic treatment of otitis media in children – comparisons with conventional therapy. International Journal of Clinical Pharmacology Therapy 35(7):296–301

Oberbaum M, Schreiber R, Rosenthal C et al 2003 Homeopathic treatment in emergency medicine: a case series. Homeopathy 92(1):44–47

### Agnus castus (Agnus castus)

Homeopathic remedy prepared from chasteberry and prescribed for physical breakdown following addictions, depressions, anxiety and fatigue, menopausal symptoms, postnatal depression and premenstrual syndrome.

Evidence:    One study suggests that a commercial preparation of agnus castus in homeopathic dilution may influence infertility in women.

Safety:    No specific information available.

Bibliography

Bergmann J, Luft B, Boehmann S et al 2000 The efficacy of the complex medication Phyto-Hypophyson L in female, hormone-related sterility: a randomized, placebo-controlled clinical double-blind study. Forschende Komplementärmedizin und Klassische Naturheilkunde 7(4):190–199

## Apis (Apis mellifera)

Remedy reflecting characteristics of irritability and nervousness with a tendency to be bossy and overprotective of their environment. Prepared from the honey bee and prescribed for insect bites and other stinging pains with swelling and itching; burning, stinging pain of urinary tract infections; used for allergic conditions, sore throat and hot stabbing, headaches.

Evidence: No specific evidence was found.

Safety: No specific information was found.

Bibliography

Berrebi A, Parant O, Ferval F et al 2001 Treatment of pain due to unwanted lactation with a homeopathic preparation given in the immediate post-partum period. Journal of Gynecology Obstetric Biological Reproduction (Paris) 30(4):353–357

Conforti A, Bellavite P, Bertani S et al 2007 Rat models of acute inflammation: a randomized controlled study on the effects of homeopathic remedies. BMC Complementary Alternative Medicine 7:1

Friese K H, Kruse S, Lüdtke R et al 1997 The homoeopathic treatment of otitis media in children – comparisons with conventional therapy. International Journal of Clinical Pharmacology Therapy 35(7):296–301

Gilruth C 1996 Apis to the rescue. Homeopathy Today 16(1):10, 12–13

Morrison R 1998 A series of apis cases. Simillimum 11(2):62–78

## Arnica (Arnica montana)

A remedy reflecting characteristics of a morbid imagination, feelings of hopelessness, with morose outlook and feelings of restlessness. Prepared from the herb Arnica montana and prescribed as a common first aid remedy for physical and emotional shock, following bereavement, accident or surgery, childbirth, sore muscles, bruises or sprains, head injury. Available as a lotion or cream although the cream should not be applied direct to open wounds.

Evidence:    No specific evidence was found.

Safety:    No specific information was found.

### Bibliography

Aris A, Gonnet N, Chaussard C et al 2008 Effect of homeopathy on analgesic intake following knee ligament reconstruction: a phase III monocentre randomized placebo controlled study. British Journal of Clinical Pharmacology 65(2):180–187

Brinkhaus B, Wilkens J M, Lüdtke R 2006 Homeopathic arnica therapy in patients receiving knee surgery: results of three randomised double-blind trials. Complementary Therapies in Medicine 14(4):237–246

Karow J H, Abt H P, Fröhling M et al 2008 Efficacy of Arnica montana D4 for healing of wounds after hallux valgus surgery compared to diclofenac. Journal of Alternative and Complementary Medicine 14(1):17–25

Kouzi S A, Nuzum D S 2007 Arnica for bruising and swelling. American Journal of Health Systems and Pharmacy 64(23):2434–2443

Robertson A, Suryanarayanan R, Banerjee A 2007 Homeopathic Arnica montana for post-tonsillectomy analgesia: a randomised placebo control trial. Homeopathy 96(1):17–21

Widrig R, Suter A, Saller R et al 2007 Choosing between NSAID and arnica for topical treatment of hand osteoarthritis in a randomised, double-blind study. Rheumatology International 27(6):585–591

## *Arsen. alb.* (Arsenicum album)

A polychrest homeopathic remedy with wide ranging application, prepared from arsenic and prescribed for insecurity and oversensitivity, general anxiety and worry, digestive disorders which cause vomiting and burning, indigestion, excess alcohol intake, asthma, mental strain and headaches with vomiting and acute inflammation.

Evidence:    May be of value in combating arsenic poisoning.

Safety:    No specific information was found.

### Bibliography

Belon P, Banerjee A, Karmakar S R et al 2007 Homeopathic remedy for arsenic toxicity? Evidence-based findings from a randomized placebo-controlled double blind human trial. Science of the Total Environment 384(1–3):141–150

Chakraborti D, Mukherjee S C, Saha K C et al 2003 Arsenic toxicity from homeopathic treatment. Clinical Toxicology 41(7):963–967

Khuda-Bukhsh A R, Pathak S, Guha B et al 2005 Can homeopathic arsenic remedy combat arsenic poisoning in humans exposed to groundwater arsenic contamination? A preliminary report on first human trial. Evidence Based Complementary Alternative Medicine 2(4):537–548

Prasad H R, Malhotra A K, Hanna N et al 2006 Arsenicosis from homeopathic medicines: a growing concern. Clinical Experimental Dermatology 31(3):497–498

## *Belladonna* (Atropa belladonna)

A constitutional remedy prepared from the deadly nightshade plant and reflecting characteristics of a very fit healthy mind, lively and entertaining personality, prone occasionally to be restless and agitated. Prescribed for acute onset of inflammatory conditions, high pyrexia with dilated pupils and delirium, throbbing headache, photophobia and symptoms including flushed hot face, trembling of the limbs or convulsions.

Evidence:   Homeopathic trials supports the use in the treatment of migraine, hot flushes and otitis media.

Safety:   No specific information was found.

### Bibliography

Balzarini A, Felisi E, Martini A et al 2000 Efficacy of homeopathic treatment of skin reactions during radiotherapy for breast cancer: a randomised, double-blind clinical trial. British Homeopathic Journal 89(1):8–12

Bordet M F, Colas A, Marijnen P 2008 Treating hot flushes in menopausal women with homeopathic treatment: results of an observational study. Homeopathy 97(1):10–15

Friese K H, Kruse S, Lüdtke R et al 1997 The homoeopathic treatment of otitis media in children – comparisons with conventional therapy. International Journal of Clinical Pharmacology Therapy 35(7):296–301

Goodyear K, Lewith G, Low J L 1998 Randomized double-blind placebo-controlled trial of homoeopathic 'proving' for Belladonna C30. Journal of the Royal Society of Medicine 91(11):579–582

Walach H, Koster H, Hennig T et al 2001 The effects of homeopathic belladonna 30CH in healthy volunteers: a randomized, double blind experiment. Journal of Psychosomatic Research 50:155–160

## *Caulophyllum* (Caulophyllum thalictroides)

A remedy prepared from the blue cohosh plant and prescribed for the shooting, cramping pains of rheumatism, to accelerate labour, for weak irregular contractions, may stimulate menstruation.

Evidence:   Case reports suggest caulophyllum affects smooth muscle particularly for induction of labour.

Safety:   Caution in late pregnancy as caulophyllum may induce labour but is not always an appropriate remedy to initiate contractions and may have the reverse effect, slowing labour or creating apparently strong uterine contractions which have no effects on cervical dilatation.

Bibliography

Beer A M, Heiliger F, Lukanov J 2000 Caulophyllum D4 to introduction of labour in premature rupture of membranes: a double-blind study confirmed by an investigation into the contraction activity of smooth muscles. Focus on Alternative and Complementary Therapies 5(1):84–85

Kistin S J, Newman A D 2007 Induction of labor with homeopathy: a case report. Journal of Midwifery and Women's Health 52(3):303–307

Martin P 2002 Homeopathic induction: beyond cimicifuga and caulophyllum. Midwifery Today with International Midwife(63):28–30

Smith C A 2003 Homoeopathy for induction of labour. Cochrane Database of Systematic Reviews(4), CD003399

### *Chamomilla* (Matricaria recutita)

A constitutional homeopathic remedy reflecting attributes of intense sensitivity, irritability and impatience, easily offended, much suppressed anger. Prepared from the German chamomile and prescribed for restlessness and insomnia, colic, low pain threshold, teething problems, occasionally in labour when the mother can 'bear it no longer'.

Evidence:    No specific evidence was found.

Safety:    No specific information was found.

Bibliography

Friese K H, Kruse S, Lüdtke R et al 1997 The homoeopathic treatment of otitis media in children: comparisons with conventional therapy. International Journal of Clinical Pharmacology Therapy 35(7):296–301

Hiwat C 1999 Anger from pain: a case of Chamomilla and its DD. Homoeopathic Links, Millennium 12(5):288–290

### *China* (China officinalis)

A constitutional, homeopathic remedy prepared from cinchona bark and reflecting characteristics of hypersensitivity, idealism and being easily offended. People for whom this remedy is applicable are very imaginative and tend to fantasize. Prescribed for nervous exhaustion and weakness resulting from pyrexia and dehydration.

Evidence:   China, alone or in combination with other homeopathic remedies, may have antioxidant and other biochemical effects.
Safety:   No specific information was found.

Bibliography

Gebhardt R 2003 Antioxidative, antiproliferative and biochemical effects in HepG2 cells of a homeopathic remedy and its constituent plant tinctures tested separately or in combination. Arzneimittelforschung 53(12):823–830

## Cimicifuga (Cimicifuga racemosa)

A constitutional, homeopathic remedy prepared from black cohosh and reflecting characteristics of excitability, extroversion, pressure of speech and flight of ideas. Prescribed primarily for disorders of menstruation, early miscarriage, childbirth, postnatal depression and the menopause.

Evidence:   Case reports indicate possible use for induction of labour.
Safety:   No information regarding safety was found, however caution in late pregnancy.

Bibliography

Martin P 2002 Homeopathic induction: beyond cimicifuga and caulophyllum. Midwifery Today with International Midwife(63):28–30

## Coffea (Coffea Arabic)

A homeopathic remedy prepared from coffee and prescribed for insomnia, excessive mental activity, extreme sensitivity to pain.

Evidence:   Animal studies suggest its effectiveness in aiding sleep onset.
Safety:   No specific information was found.

Bibliography

Ruiz-Vega G, Pérez-Ordaz L, Cortés-Galván L et al 2003 A kinetic approach to caffeine: Coffea cruda interaction. Homeopathy 92(1):19–29
Ruiz-Vega G, Pérez-Ordaz L, León-Huéramo O et al 2002 Comparative effect of Coffea cruda potencies on rats. Homeopathy 91(2):80–84

## Digitalis (Digitalis purpurea)

A homeopathic remedy prepared from the foxglove prescribed for bradycardia, heart failure, nausea at the sight of food.

Evidence:   Animal studies have demonstrated cardiac effects and reversal of adverse induced cardiac activity.

Safety:   No specific information was found.

Bibliography

Varshney J P, Chaudhuri S 2007 Atrial paroxysmal tachycardia in dogs and its management with homeopathic Digitalis: two case reports. Homeopathy 96(4):270–272

*Gelsemium* (Gelsemium sempervirens)

A constitutional, homeopathic remedy derived from yellow jasmine and reflecting characteristics of weakness and cowardice, fears and phobias. Prescribed for colds and influenza, headaches, anticipatory anxiety, i.e. stage fright or pre-examination nervousness, muscular weakness and sore throat.

Evidence:   Review articles suggest a use for stress anxiety and fatigue, although none are particularly recent publications.

Safety:   No specific information was found.

Bibliography

Kokelenberg G 1996 Chronic fatigue syndrome: a case of Gelsemium. Homoeopathic Links 9(3):153–154
Kokelenberg G 1996 Stress management problems: a case of Gelsemium. Homoeopathic Links 9(3):154–155
Miller A 1999 Fantastic for 'flu, essential for exams: getting to Gelsemium through the rubrics of the mind. Homoeopath 73:8–13

*Graphites* (Graphite)

A polychrest, constitutional, homeopathic remedy with wide-ranging application. Prepared from graphite, a form of carbon and reflecting characteristics of indecision, timidity, anxiety and lack of mental effort. Prescribed for dry, itching skin conditions such as eczema, psoriasis and keloid scars, digestive upsets and scanty menstruation.

Evidence:   Case reports suggest use in dermatological conditions.

Safety:   No information regarding safety and no evidence of contraindications was found.

Bibliography

Gupta R, Manchanda R K, Arya B S 2007 Homoeopathy for the treatment of lichen simplex chronicus: a case series. Homeopathy 96(2):139

Jones A 1998 A case of graphites in eczema. Homoeopathy (48):28–31

## Hamamelis (Hamamelis virginiana)

Remedy prepared from witch hazel and prescribed for circulatory disorders particularly chilblains and haemorrhoids, bruising, epistaxis and some forms of depression.

Evidence:   No specific evidence was found.

Safety:   No specific information was found.

Bibliography

Conforti A, Bellavite P, Bertani S et al 2007 Rat models of acute inflammation: a randomized controlled study on the effects of homeopathic remedies. BMC Complementary and Alternative Medicine 7:1

## Hypericum (Hypericum perforatum)

A remedy prepared from the herb St John's wort and prescribed for wound care, neuritis, puncture or crush injuries, back pain and depression.

Evidence:   No specific evidence found.

Safety:   No specific information available. However, care should be taken that patients are using the homeopathic dilution and not the herbal variety of remedy.

Bibliography

Paris A, Gonnet N, Chaussard C et al 2008 Effect of homeopathy on analgesic intake following knee ligament reconstruction: a phase III monocentre randomized placebo controlled study. British Journal of Clinical Pharmacology 65(2):180–187

## Ipecacuanha (Cephaelis ipecacuanha)

A remedy prepared from the root of the *Cephaelis ipecacuanha* plant and is prescribed predominantly for nausea and vomiting but may also be used for difficulty in breathing. Patients are often ill as a result of bottling up their feelings.

Evidence:   No specific clinical studies were found although some papers on veterinary use of ipecacuanha were discovered.

Safety:    No specific information was found.

Bibliography

Varshney J P, Naresh R 2004 Evaluation of a homeopathic complex in the clinical management of udder diseases of riverine buffaloes. Homeopathy 93(1): 17–20

Varshney J P, Naresh R 2005 Comparative efficacy of homeopathic and allopathic systems of medicine in the management of clinical mastitis of Indian dairy cows. Homeopathy 94(2):81–85

## *Kali. bich.* (Kalium bichromium)

A constitutional homeopathic remedy reflecting attributes of conformity, morality, rigidity and pragmatism. Prepared from potassium bichromate and prescribed for mucous membrane conditions, particularly ear, nose and throat problems such as catarrh, sinusitis and glue ear, also useful for peptic ulcer.

Evidence:    Case reports suggest use in otitis media and skin conditions.

Safety:    No information regarding safety, and no evidence of contraindications was found.

Bibliography

Friese K H, Kruse S, Lüdtke R 1997 The homoeopathic treatment of otitis media in children: comparisons with conventional therapy. International Journal of Clinical Pharmacology and Therapeutics 35(7):296–301

Gupta R, Manchanda R K, Arya B S 2007 Homoeopathy for the treatment of lichen simplex chronicus: a case series. Homeopathy 96(2):139

## *Lachesis* (Lachesis muta)

A polychrest homeopathic remedy with wide ranging applications, prepared from the venom of the bushmaster snake and prescribed for disorders of the circulatory and vascular system including palpitations and angina. Also used for wounds that are slow to heal and for gynaecological conditions particularly related to the menopause.

Evidence:    Recent research suggests a use for menopausal symptoms.

Safety:    No specific information was found.

Bibliography

Bordet M F, Colas A, Marijnen P et al 2008 Treating hot flushes in menopausal women with homeopathic treatment: results of an observational study. Homeopathy 97(1):10–15

## *Lycopodium* (Lycopodium clavatum)

A constitutional, polychrest homeopathic remedy with wide ranging applications, prepared from a plant known as club moss or wolf's claws and reflecting characteristics of quiet self-possession, stability and detachment, intellectual and conservative. Prescribed for digestive disorders, urinary tract problems and emotional problems caused by insecurity and self consciousness.

Evidence: There is some suggestion that lycopodium, with other homeopathic remedies, may have anti-cancer properties although the mechanism of action is not yet understood.

Safety: No specific information was found.

Bibliography

Kumar K B, Sunila E S, Kuttan G et al 2007 Inhibition of chemically induced carcinogenesis by drugs used in homeopathic medicine. Asian Pacific Journal of Cancer Prevention 8(1):98–102
Rajendran E S 2004 Homeopathy as a supportive therapy in cancer. Homeopathy 93(2):99–102

## *Nat. mur.* (Natrum muriaticum)

A constitutional, polychrest homeopathic remedy with wide ranging applications, prepared from common salt or sodium chloride and reflecting characteristics of refinement and sensitivity, easily hurt by criticism or insults. Prescribed for emotional problems such as anxiety and depression resulting from suppressed feelings or denial. Also used for colds and catarrh and headaches related to menstruation and premenstrual syndrome.

Evidence: No specific evidence was found.

Safety: No specific information was found.

Bibliography

Becker-Witt C, Lüdtke R, Weisshuhn T E et al 2004 Diagnoses and treatment in homeopathic medical practice. Forschende Komplementärmedizin und Klassische Naturheilkunde 11(2):98–103

### Nux vomica (Strychnos nux vomica)

A polychrest homeopathic remedy with wide ranging application, prepared from the seeds of the poison nut tree and prescribed for general tension from anger, frustration and mental strain to insomnia and digestive upsets. Also used for cardiovascular problems caused by nervous tension.

Evidence:   Possible use for gastrointestinal conditions.

Safety:   No information regarding safety and no evidence of contraindications was found.

Bibliography

Gupta R, Manchanda R K 2006 Reiter's disease treated with Nux vomica. Homeopathy 95(2):103–104
Jones A 1999 Homoeopathic case studies: Nux vomica for bowel symptoms. Positive Health 37:25
Sukul A, Sarkar P, Sinhababu S P et al 2000 Altered solution structure of alcoholic medium of potentized Nux vomica underlies its antialcoholic effect. British Homeopathic Journal 89(2):73–77

### Opium (Papaver somniferum)

A remedy prepared from the opium poppy and prescribed for two mental states following severe fright or shock presenting as over-excitement or denial. Useful for alcohol withdrawal.

Evidence:   One paper reported its use in a neonatal emergency.

Safety:   No specific information was found.

Bibliography

Bauer J 2006 Attacks of apnea in a newborn aged 18 days. Forschende Komplementärmedizin 13(4):241–243
Oberbaum M, Schreiber R, Rosenthal C et al 2003 Homeopathic treatment in emergency medicine: a case series. Homeopathy 92(1):44–47

*Petroleum* (Oleum petrae)

A remedy prepared from petroleum, prescribed for skin conditions, dry eczema, nausea and vomiting, particularly travel sickness.

Evidence:    No specific evidence was found.

Safety:    No specific information was found.

### Bibliography

Gnaiger-Rathmanner J, Schneider A, Loader B et al 2008 Petroleum: a series of 25 cases. Homeopathy 97(2):83–88

*Pulsatilla* (Pulsatilla nigricans)

A constitutional, polychrest homeopathic remedy prepared from the windflower, reflecting characteristics of a sweet nature, shy kind and gentle people who tend to be dependant on others and accepting of guidance and advice. Pulsatilla also has the characteristics of change, so it is useful for those who keep vacillating and are unable to make decisions. Commonly, pulsatilla-types are fair-haired female patients. Prescribed for digestive conditions resulting from over-indulgence, especially rich fatty foods, depression and menstrual disorders and other gynaecological problems.

Evidence:    Animal studies have shown its use in infertility and conception; clinical case reports of use for respiratory conditions are also available.

Safety:    No specific information was found.

### Bibliography

Colin P 2006 Homeopathy and respiratory allergies: a series of 147 cases. Homeopathy 95(2):68–72

Friese K H, Kruse S, Lüdtke R et al 1997 The homoeopathic treatment of otitis media in children: comparisons with conventional therapy. International Journal of Clinical Pharmacology and Therapeutics 35(7):296–301

Lobreiro J 2007 Homeopathic treatment for infertility in a prize Nelore bull. Homeopathy 96(1):49–51

Rajkumar R, Srivastava S K, Yadav M C et al 2006 Effect of a Homeopathic complex on oestrus induction and hormonal profile in anoestrus cows. Homeopathy 95(3):131–135

*Rhus tox.* (Rhus toxicodendron)

A constitutional homeopathic remedy reflecting characteristics of cheerful liveliness, witty, hard working but easily frustrated, prepared from the poison ivy plant and prescribed for red, itchy skin complaints, rheumatic type pain joints and muscles, menorrhagia and depression.

Evidence:   Inconclusive.

Safety:   No specific information was found.

### Bibliography

Abbot N C 1997 Homoeopathic Arnica and Rhus tox do not help muscle soreness. FACT 2(2):62–63

dos Santos A L, Perazzo F F, Cardoso L G et al 2007 In vivo study of the antiinflammatory effect of Rhus toxicodendron. Homeopathy 96(2):95–101

*Sepia* (Sepia officinalis)

A constitutional, polychrest homeopathic remedy with wide ranging applications, prepared from the ink of the cuttle fish and reflecting characteristics of imposed martyrdom and feeling overwhelmed by life's demands and very resentful. Prescribed for gynaecological problems, PMS, dyspareunia and is one of the principle remedies for postnatal depression.

Evidence:   No specific evidence was found.

Safety:   No specific information was found.

### Bibliography

Bordet M F, Colas A, Marijnen P et al 2008 Treating hot flushes in menopausal women with homeopathic treatment: results of an observational study. Homeopathy 97(1):10–15

*Thuja* (Thuja occidentalis)

A constitutional, polychrest homeopathic remedy reflecting characteristics of low self esteem, poor self image and depression and having a wide ranging application. Prepared from the conifer tree or arbour vitae (tree of life) and prescribed, depending on presenting symptoms, for: dermatological conditions, urethral and vaginal infections, loss of appetite and stress-related headaches.

Evidence: There is some emerging suggestion that thuja and other homeopathic remedies may be protective against certain cancers.

Safety: No specific information was found.

### Bibliography

Kumar K B, Sunila E S, Kuttan G et al 2007 Inhibition of chemically induced carcinogenesis by drugs used in homeopathic medicine. Asian Pacific Journal of Cancer Prevention 8(1):98–102

## Hypnosis/hypnotherapy

*Description*

Hypnosis is traditionally regarded as an altered state of consciousness, similar to the state of absorption experienced when listening to music, watching television, day dreaming or concentrating on a task. When used as a clinical intervention, the hypnotic state is induced by the therapist using techniques such as progressive relaxation and guided image. The state of hypnosis is associated with an increased degree of suggestibility, facilitating an interaction between the hypnotherapist and the subject, allowing the practitioner to make suggestions to facilitate the person to alter the way he or she thinks, feels or reacts to certain events or situations. The hypnotic 'trance' is defined as focused attention, dis-attention to extraneous stimuli and absorption in some image or thought. Effectiveness of the therapy is only weakly related to hypnotizability, although measuring instruments have been devised notably the Stanford Hypnotic Clinical Scale for Adults.

Evidence: Clinical trials support the use of hypnosis in any condition which is exacerbated by psycho-emotional issues, including stress, anxiety, fear and tension. There is a growing body of clinical evidence for the effectiveness of hypnotherapy for depression, asthma, childbirth preparation, enuresis, pain relief, eating disorders and irritable bowel syndrome.

Safety: Hypnosis is a naturally occurring phenomenon and is not intrinsically dangerous but its application by poorly or untrained therapists can cause problems, as sensationalized by the media occasionally. Deep relaxation is contraindicated in acute psychotic states or those susceptible to psychosis, trance-like states can lead to feelings of disorientation and depersonalization and should not be entered into for long periods. Deep relaxation may induce seizures in susceptible patients. Emotional abreaction may occur.

## Bibliography

Alladin A, Alibahal S 2007 Cognitive hypnotherapy for depression: an empirical investigation. International Journal of Clinical and Experimental Hypnosis 55(2):147–166

Barabasz M 2007 Efficacy of hypnotherapy in the treatment of eating disorders. International Journal of Clinical and Experimental Hypnosis 55(3): 318–335

Brown D 2007 Evidence based hypnotherapy for asthma: a critical review. International Journal of Clinical and Experimental Hypnosis 55(2): 220–249

Brown D C, Hammond D C 2007 Evidence-based clinical hypnosis for obstetrics, labor and delivery and preterm labor. International Journal of Clinical and Experimental Hypnosis 55(3):355–371

Elkins G, Jensen M, Patterson D 2007 Hypnotherapy for the management of chronic pain. International Journal of Clinical and Experimental Hypnosis 55(3):275–287

Gholamrezaei A, Ardestani S, Emami M 2006 Where does hypnotherapy stand in the management of irritable bowel syndrome? A systematic review. Journal of Alternative Complementary Medicine 12(6):517–527

Graci G, Hardie J 2007 Evidence based hypnotherapy for the management of sleep disorders. International Journal of Clinical and Experimental Hypnosis 55(3):288–302

Iglesias A, Iglesias A 2008 Secondary diurnal enuresis treated with hypnosis: a time-series design. International Journal of Clinical and Experimental Hypnosis 56(2):229–240

Jensen M, McArthur K, Barber J et al 2006 Satisfaction with and beneficial side-effects of hypnotic analgesia. International Journal of Clinical and Experimental Hypnosis 54(4):432–447

Jensen M P, Barber J, Hanley M A et al 2008 Long-term outcome of hypnotic-analgesia treatment for chronic pain in persons with disabilities. International Journal of Clinical and Experimental Hypnosis 56(2):156–169

Jensen M P, Barber J, Hanley M A et al 2008 Long-term outcome of hypnotic-analgesia treatment for chronic pain in persons with disabilities. International Journal of Clinical and Experimental Hypnosis 56(2):156–169

Kuijpers H J, van der Heijden F M, Tuinier S et al 2007 Meditation-induced psychosis. Psychopathology 40(6):461–464

Marc I, Rainville P, Dodin S 2008 Hypnotic induction and therapeutic suggestions in first-trimester pregnancy termination. International Journal of Clinical and Experimental Hypnosis 56(2):214–228

Olson D M, Howard N, Shaw R J 2008 Hypnosis-provoked nonepileptic events in children. Epilepsy Behavior 12(3):456–459

Shakibaei F, Harandi A A, Gholamrezaei A et al 2008 Hypnotherapy in management of pain and reexperiencing of trauma in burn patients. International Journal of Clinical and Experimental Hypnosis 56(2):185–197

Yexley M 2007 Treating postpartum depression with hypnosis: addressing specific symptoms presented by the client. American Journal of Clinical Hypnosis 49(3):219–223

### Resources

The British Society of Clinical and Academic Hypnosis: www.bscah.org

## Guided visualization/imagery

*Description*

Guided imagery may be used alone or in conjunction with hypnosis and engages the mind to imagine a variety of scenarios, either as a diagnostic technique or as a direct healing intervention. Scenarios and images may be selected by the patient before the session starts or developed by the therapist during the session.

Evidence: Some evidence supports the use of guided imagery in reducing stress and improving quality of life. As a stand-alone relaxation technique it has been used to reduce stress and anxiety in patients with cancer, and particularly with the elderly.

Safety:  No specific safety information was found.

### Bibliography

Crow S, Banks D 2004 Guided imagery: a tool to guide the way for the nursing home patient. Advances Mind-Body Medicine 20(4):4–7

Menzies V, Gill Taylor A 2004 The idea of imagination: an analysis of 'imagery'. Advances in Mind-Body Medicine 20(2):4–10

Nunes D F, Rodriguez A L, da Silva Hoffmann F et al 2007 Relaxation and guided imagery program in patients with breast cancer undergoing radiotherapy is not associated with neuroimmunomodulatory effects. Journal of Psychosomatic Research 63(6):647–655

Paddock J R, Terranova S 2001 Guided visualization and suggestibility: effect of perceived authority on recall of autobiographical memories. Journal of Genetic Psychology 162(3):347–356

Sharpe P A, Williams H G, Granner M L et al 2007 A randomised study of the effects of massage therapy compared to guided relaxation on well-being and stress perception among older adults. Complementary Therapies in Medicine 15(3):157–163

# N

## Naturopathy/naturopathic medicine

*Description*

The foundation and development of naturopathy is credited to Benedick Lust who bought the patent to the name 'naturopathy' in 1902 to describe an eclectic system of healthcare which, today, encompasses a range of interventions including dietary reform, exercise, homeopathy, osteopathy, chiropractic and herbal medicine. The original form of naturopathy arose from a combination of the nature cure movement, which is based on a vegetarian diet combined with light, air and therapeutic baths and the Hygienic movement, which encourages consumption of raw vegetarian, food and freshly squeezed juices in the correct combinations to maximize digestion. The philosophy behind naturopathy includes the concept of the healing power of nature, the inherent ability of the body to heal itself and the concept of constitutional types related to the five elements of water, fire, earth, wood and metal. The human body is viewed as consisting of mechanical, mental/emotional and chemical parts in equal proportions (called the healing triad), which are taken into account during diagnosis and therapy. Techniques used to aid diagnosis include history-taking, iridology, face, tongue, temple or skull diagnosis and Hara diagnosis, based on examination of the pulses and abdomen.

## Hydrotherapy/balneotherapy

*Description*

Balneotherapy is a key component of naturopathy and includes: steam baths, whirlpool baths to provide underwater massage, foot baths; sitz baths, in which the patient alternately immerses their hips in cold and feet in hot water, respectively, alternating the positions during the treatment; blitz gus, in which a jet of water is directed at the patient from a distance of between 25–50 feet; cold friction rub, in which a coarse washcloth is dipped in cold water and rubbed vigorously across the body as a tonifying treatment; a cold immersion bath, for which patients are immersed for 4–20 min in a temperature of 10–23 °C to stimulate circulation and the central nervous system and to reduce pyrexia; a graduated bath, when patients are immersed in a bath at 31 °C and the temperature is slowly lowered at 1 °C/hour to a temperature of 25 °C to reduce pyrexia, for a general tonic effect and to energize the heart; a hip bath to relieve pelvic pain, congestion and genitourinary conditions; and a hot full immersion bath which involves soaking the whole body in water at 40–45 °C to cleanse the body, relax muscles and induce sweating. Wet sheet treatments are also used, in which the patient is wrapped in cold wet sheets and covered with blankets and left until they begin to sweat, at which point, the blankets are removed and the patient drenched with cold water.

Evidence: Case reports and some clinical studies suggest a role for naturopathy for arthritis, menopausal symptoms and pain relief.

Safety: Pregnant women, children and the elderly, and patients with hypertension, hypotension and cardiac conditions should avoid steam or hot baths unless prescribed by an appropriately qualified practitioner; care must be taken regarding temperature control to avoid scalding.

Bibliography

Dunn J M, Wilkinson J M 2005 Naturopathic management of rheumatoid arthritis. Modern Rheumatology 15(2):87–90

Forestier R, Françon A 2008 Crenobalneotherapy for limb osteoarthritis: systematic literature review and methodological analysis. Joint, Bone, Spine 75(2):138–148

Greenlee H, Atkinson C, Stanczyk F Z et al 2007 A pilot and feasibility study on the effects of naturopathic botanical and dietary interventions on sex steroid hormone metabolism in premenopausal women. Cancer Epidemiology, Biomarkers and Prevention 16(8):1601–1609

Gupta P J 2008 Warm sitz bath does not reduce symptoms in posthaemorrhoidectomy period: a randomized, controlled study. ANZ Journal of Surgery 78(5):398–401

Gupta P 2006 Randomized, controlled study comparing sitz-bath and no-sitz-bath treatments in patients with acute anal fissures. ANZ Journal of Surgery 76(8): 718–721

Herman P M, Szczurko O, Cooley K et al 2008 Cost-effectiveness of naturopathic care for chronic low back pain. Alternative Therapies in Health and Medicine 14(2):32–39

Liao W C, Landis C A, Lentz M J et al 2005 Effect of foot bathing on distal-proximal skin temperature gradient in elders. International Journal of Nursing Studies 42(7):717–722

Short R W, Agredano Y Z, Choi J M et al 2008 A single-blinded, randomized pilot study to evaluate the effect of exercise-induced sweat on truncal acne. Pediatric Dermatology 25(1):126–128

Vaht M, Birkenfeldt R, Ubner M 2008 An evaluation of the effect of differing lengths of spa therapy upon patients with osteoarthritis (OA). Complementary Therapies in Clinical Practice 14(1):60–64

Verhagen A, Bierma-Zeinstra S, Lambeck J et al 2008 Balneotherapy for osteoarthritis. A Cochrane review. Journal of Rheumatology 35(6):1118–1123

Weber W, Taylor J A, McCarty R L et al 2007 Frequency and characteristics of pediatric and adolescent visits in naturopathic medical practice. Pediatrics 120(1):e142–e146

### Resources

British Naturopathy Association: www.naturopaths.org.uk
General Council and Register of Naturopaths: www.naturopathy.org.uk

## Nutritional therapies

*Description*

The role of food as a form of medicine has long been recognized. Nutritional therapy can be a therapy in its own right but is also an integral part of naturopathy and many other forms of complementary and alternative medicine (see also Naturopathy and Cancer Therapies sections). The therapeutic use of food is based on the understanding that modern diets are poor in nutrients due to over-farming, climatic changes and environmental issues and that individuals have different nutritional requirements, according to age, gender, lifestyle and health. Nutritional therapy differs from conventional dietetics in that, in the latter, dietary changes are required to deal with the effects of the disease process, as in diabetes mellitus, whereas nutritional therapy focuses on poor nutrition as a cause of ill-health. It is thought that in disease resulting from poor nutrition, specific nutrients and dietary manipulation can prove a potent means of restoring nutritional balance and, ultimately, good health. Nutritional therapists use a range of diagnostic tests for deficiencies or allergies before prescribing a dietary regimen to suit the patient.

Evidence:    There is considerable evidence regarding the uses and safety issues related to nutritional therapies. However, most references are specific to the dietary regimen, therefore a limited selections of generic references have been included here.

Safety: It is possible that radical dietary changes may trigger other health problems and lead to nutritional deficiencies and delay in seeking appropriate medical advice. Vulnerable people should be advised to ensure that the practitioner is adequately registered and maintains a communication channel with conventional healthcare professionals, where appropriate, e.g. children, adolescents, pregnant and lactating mothers and the elderly.

### Bibliography

Clifton P M, Keogh J 2007 Metabolic effects of high-protein diets. Current Atherosclerosis Reports 9(6):472–478

Gura K M, Lee S, Valim C et al 2008 Safety and efficacy of a fish-oil-based fat emulsion in the treatment of parenteral nutrition-associated liver disease. Pediatrics 121(3):e678–e686

Hollander J M, Mechanick J I 2008 Complementary and alternative medicine and the management of the metabolic syndrome. Journal of the American Diet Association 108(3):495–509

Lucey A J, Paschos G K, Cashman K D et al 2008 Influence of moderate energy restriction and seafood consumption on bone turnover in overweight young adults. American Journal of Clinical Nutrition 87(4):1045–1052

Samaha F F, Foster G D, Makris A P 2007 Low-carbohydrate diets, obesity and metabolic risk factors for cardiovascular disease. Current Atherosclerosis Reports 9(6):441–447

Wernerman J 2008 Role of glutamine supplementation in critically ill patients. Current Opinion in Anaesthesiology 21(2):155–159

### Resources

British Association of Nutritional Therapy (BANT): www.bant.org.uk
The Nutritional Therapy Council: www.nutritionaltherapycouncil.org.uk

## Apitherapy

*Description*

Apitherapy is the medicinal use of various products of *Apis mellifera*, the common honey bee.

Bee venom uses the bee sting for its antiinflammatory properties and is traditionally used to treat rheumatoid arthritis, bursitis and tendonitis. In traditional Chinese medicine it is injected into acupuncture points to treat collagen-induced arthritis. Bee venom contains melittin, which has strong antiinflammatory and short-acting histaminic effects; peptide 401 mast cell degenerating protein, which reduces inflammation and pain through local action on tissue inflammation; and phospholipase A which emulsifies debris within the joints and other tissues.

Bee pollen, which contains proteins, carbohydrates, minerals, vitamins and essential fatty acids, is formed from flower pollen and nectar mixed with saliva from the worker honey bees and is traditionally used for allergies, asthma, reducing cholesterol, hypertension and prostatic hypertrophy.

Honey contains hydrogen peroxide, formed by the enzyme glucose oxidase which is broken down partly by the catalase enzyme present in all body tissues and serum. Manuka honey, in particular, is a valuable aid to wound care and is produced commercially, sterilized and packaged for medicinal use. Propolis or 'bee glue' is the resinous product collected by the honey bee from plants and trees and, when mixed with saliva and wax, is used to repair and strengthen the inner surfaces of their hives; it may to also act as an antimicrobial within the hive and is traditionally used as an antifungal, antibacterial and inflammatory agent and in wound healing. Propolis contains phenolic compounds, flavonoids, pinobanksin and pinobanksin 3-acetate, thought to be responsible for the antibacterial, antifungal, antiviral and immunostimulant properties, together with beeswax, resins vitamins and amino acids.

Royal jelly is created by the worker bee and fed to the queen bee. It is traditionally used as a treatment for: sexual dysfunction, baldness, menopause and disease prevention. Royal jelly contains 70% water, with small amounts of proteins, carbohydrates, fats, vitamins and minerals, amino acids and gammaglobulin.

Evidence:   Bee venom has been shown to help arthritis and multiple sclerosis. Honey has strong wound healing properties and is effective in combating infection including *Staphylococcus aureus*, *Escherichia coli*, *Streptococcus pyogenes*, *Helicobacter* and *Candida albicans*. Manuka honey has been used to combat MRSA. Royal jelly appears to have hyperglycaemic and hypocholesterolaemic effects.

Safety:   Be aware of known or suspected allergy to bee products. Honey used therapeutically in wound dressings should be sterilized, as unsterilized honey may contain *Clostridium botulinum*. Honey available for public consumption is generally pasteurized, a process which does not kill the spores. Royal jelly is contraindicated in asthmatics; death has been reported following bronchospasm after ingesting royal jelly; it may also interact with anticoagulants, particularly warfarin.

### Bibliography

Blaser G 2007 Effect of medical honey on wounds colonised or infected with MRSA. Journal of Wound Care 16(8):325–328

Couteau C, Pommier M, Paparis E 2008 Photo-protective activity of propolis. Natural Product Research 22(3):264–268

Gasic S, Vucevic D, Vasilijic S et al 2007 Evaluation of the immunomodulatory activities of royal jelly components in vitro. Immunopharmacology Immunotoxicology 29(3–4):521–536

Guo H, Saiga A, Sato M et al 2007 Royal jelly supplementation improves lipoprotein metabolism in humans. Journal of Nutritional Science and Vitaminology 53(4):345–348

Lee N, Fermo J 2006 Warfarin and royal jelly interaction. Pharmacotherapy 26(4):583–586

Lee J, Kim S, Kim T et al 2004 Antiinflammatory effects of bee venom on type II collagen induced arthritis. American Journal of Chinese Medicine 32(3): 361–367

Mullai V, Menon T 2007 Bactericidal activity of different types of honey against clinical and environmental isolates of Pseudomonas aeruginosa. Journal of Alternative and Complementary Medicine 13(4):439–441

Sforcin J 2007 Propolis and the immune system: a review. Journal of Ethnopharmacology 113(1):1–14

Takahama H, Shimazu T 2006 Food induced anaphylaxis caused by ingestion of royal jelly. Journal of Dermatology 33(6):424–426

Testi S, Cecchi L, Severino M et al 2007 Severe anaphylaxis to royal jelly attributed to cefonicid. Journal of Investigative Allergology Clinical Immunology 17(4):281

Velazquez C, Navarro M, Acosta A et al 2007 Antibacterial and free radical scavenging activities of Sonoran propolis. Journal of Applied Microbiology 103(5):1747–1756

Wesselius T, Heersema D, Mostert J 2005 A randomised cross over study for bee sting therapy for multiple sclerosis. Neurology 65(11):1764–1768

# Blue–green algae (*Spirulina*)

*Description*

Blue–green algae is a nutritional supplement containing 65–70% protein, high concentrations of vitamin B, iron and other minerals. It is thought to be hypoglycaemic, antiviral and to act as a tonic.

Evidence:   Clinical trials support its use as an antiinflammatory. Trials are currently investigating its potential in a variety of diseases, including malnourishment in children with HIV.

Safety:   Blue–green algae may be harvested in uncontrolled settings and there is risk of contamination with heavy metals, including mercury. It can contain high levels of phenylalanine, which may cause adverse reactions in people with phenylketonuria and should be used with caution. It should be avoided during pregnancy and breast-feeding.

---

## Bibliography

Baicus C, Baicus A 2007 Spirulina did not ameliorate idiopathic chronic fatigue in four N-of-1 randomized controlled trials. Phytotherapy Research 21(6): 570–573

Kraigher O, Wohl Y, Gat A et al 2008 A mixed immunoblistering disorder exhibiting features of bullous pemphigoid and pemphigus foliaceus associated with Spirulina algae intake. International Journal of Dermatology 47(1):61–63

Lu H K, Hsieh C C, Hsu J J et al 2006 Preventive effects of Spirulina platensis on skeletal muscle damage under exercise-induced oxidative stress. European Journal of Applied Physiology 98(2):220–226

Mao T K, Van de Water J, Gershwin M E 2005 Effects of a Spirulina-based dietary supplement on cytokine production from allergic rhinitis patients. Journal of Medicinal Food 8(1):27–30

McCarty M F 2007 Clinical potential of Spirulina as a source of phycocyanobilin. Journal of Medicinal Food 10(4):566–570

Samuels R, Mani U V, Iyer U M et al 2002 Hypocholesterolemic effect of spirulina in patients with hyperlipidemic nephrotic syndrome. Journal of Medicinal Food 5(2):91–96

Simpore J, Zongo F, Kabore F et al 2005 Nutrition rehabilitation of HIV-infected and HIV-negative undernourished children utilizing spirulina. Annals of Nutrition and Metabolism 49(6):373–380

Shyam R, Singh S, Vats P 2007 Wheat grass supplementation decreases oxidative stress in health subjects: comparison study with spirulina. Journal of Alternative and Complementary Medicine 13(8):789–791

Thakur S, Pushpakumara B 2007 Influence of spirulina on the phenytoin induced haematological changes. Ancient Science of Life 26(3–4):9–15

Vitale S, Miller L, Mejico J et al 2004 A randomized placebo controlled crossover clinical trial of super blue-green algae in patients with essential blepharospasm or Meige syndrome. American Journal of Ophthalmology 138(1):18–32

## Chicken soup

*Description*

Chicken soup is a folk remedy used as a cold remedy since the 12th century and has recently been recognized as having several antiinflammatory properties, which are particularly valuable in treating respiratory tract infections.

Evidence: No clinical trials could be found although there is some interest among conventional healthcare professionals in the potential value of chicken soup; however, any reported benefits may be a placebo effect.

Safety: No specific safety information was found.

Bibliography

Hopkins A B 2003 Chicken soup cure may not be a myth. Nurse Practitioner 28(6):16

Jefferson T 2002 Advances in the diagnosis and management of influenza. Current Infectious Diseases Reports 4(3):206–210

Lavine J B 2001 Chicken soup or Jewish medicine. Chest 119(4):1295

Nagatsuka N, Harada K, Ando M et al 2006 Measurement of the radical scavenging activity of chicken jelly soup, a part of the medicated diet, 'Yakuzen', made from gelatin gel food 'Nikogori', using chemiluminescence and electron spin resonance methods. International Journal of Molecular Medicine 18(1):107–111

Schaffner M 2004 Leading the way: chicken soup for the certifying soul. Gastroenterology Nursing 27(2):76–77.

## Co-enzyme Q-10

*Description*

Co-enzyme Q-10 is a nutritional supplement consisting of a naturally occurring enzyme found in the mitochondria of body cells, which is important for energy production in cells and a free radical scavenger and antioxidant. It is found naturally in oily fish such as sardines, mackerel, whole grain cereals, soya beans, meat and poultry but is now also available as commercially produced supplements.

Evidence: Case reports and some clinical studies support the use of co-enzyme Q-10 in myocardial rehabilitation; it has been shown to be antiinflammatory and hypotensive.

Safety: Not to be used in cardiovascular disease without supervision. May diminish responses to warfarin, whereas oral anti-diabetic drugs may reduce the purported effects of co-enzyme Q10 and vitamin E may reduce blood levels of co-enzyme Q10. It is thought to be hypotensive so should be used with caution in those with pathological variations in blood pressure. If taken as a supplement, it should not be taken in doses higher than those recommended by the manufacturer, nor for prolonged periods of time.

### Bibliography

Burke B, Neuenschwander R, Olson R 2001 Randomized double blind placebo controlled trial of co-enzyme Q10 in isolated systolic hypertension. Southern Medical Journal 94(11):1112–1117

Gvozdjáková A, Kucharská J, Bartkovjaková M 2005 Coenzyme Q10 supplementation reduces corticosteroids dosage in patients with bronchial asthma. Biofactors 25(1–4):235–240

Hadj A, Esmore D, Rowland M 2006 Pre-operative preparation for cardiac surgery utilising a combination of metabolic, physical and mental therapy. Heart Lung Circular 15(3):172–181

Jones K, Hughes K, Mischley L et al 2004 Coenzyme Q-10 and cardiovascular health. Alternative Therapies in Health and Medicine 10(1):22–30

Müller T, Büttner T, Gholipour A F et al 2003 Coenzyme Q10 supplementation provides mild symptomatic benefit in patients with Parkinson's disease. Neuroscience Letters 341(3):201–204

Richard C L, Jurgens T M 2005 Effects of natural health products on blood pressure. Annals of Pharmacotherapy 39(4):712–720

Rodriguez M C, MacDonald J R, Mahoney D J 2007 Beneficial effects of creatine, CoQ10 and lipoic acid in mitochondrial disorders. Muscle and Nerve 35(2):235–242

Tang P H, Miles M V, Steele P et al 2002 Anticoagulant effects on plasma coenzyme Q(10) estimated by HPLC with coulometric detection. Clinica Chimica Acta 318(1–2):127–131

## Detoxification

*Description*

Detoxification is a concept germane to several complementary and alternative interventions and involves the removal of accumulated substances from the body which are perceived as harmful. The process usually includes a period of fasting followed by a restricted diet for a number of days or weeks and the ingestion of detoxifying herbs or other products. The regimen may include colonic irrigation.

Evidence:    There is no evidence of any need for detoxification in the normal way, with the exception of drugs, alcohol and in rare instances heavy metals which should be conducted under medical supervision. It has been shown that some people react to certain additives in their food and these can be avoided without excessive disruption to the diet.

Safety:    Side-effects include headache, weakness, irritability and light-headedness. Although 'toxins' are claimed to have an adverse effect on the body, except for the occasional incidence of heavy metal poisoning, the body is perfectly capable of dealing with them through the normal detoxification and excretory routes. If, for any reason, an excretory organ is not functioning properly the patient needs to be referred to a medical practitioner. Detoxification is contraindicated in pregnant women, diabetics, children and patients with eating disorders.

### Bibliography

Jeffery E H 2007 Detoxification basics. Alternative Therapies in Health and Medicine 13(2):S96–S97

Minich D M, Bland J S 2007 Acid-alkaline balance: role in chronic disease and detoxification. Alternative Therapies in Health and Medicine 13(4):62–65

Weitzman S 2008 Complementary and alternative (CAM) dietary therapies for cancer. Pediatric Blood Cancer 50(Suppl):494–497

## Fasting

### Description

Fasting is a therapeutic procedure to facilitate elimination of toxins and promote healing in the belief that it helps to cleanse the liver and kidneys, purify the blood and enhance the immune system. There is usually a preparatory period during which only fruit and vegetables are consumed, followed by either a water-only fast or a modified form in which juices, fruit or vegetables are allowed (e.g. the grape cancer fast), varying in length from 1 to 15 days. Food is then reintroduced gradually in small portions.

Evidence:    There is some evidence that short-term, supervised fasting may have some benefits.

Safety:    Prolonged unsupervised fasting may impair the immune system rather than enhance it, by depriving the body of essential nutrients, resulting in electrolyte imbalances and the possibility of cardiac arrhythmias and hypotension. Side-effects include nausea, headaches, mucus production, weakness and muscle catabolism, which have previously been considered to be due to toxins being eliminated. Contraindicated in pregnant and lactating women, children, diabetics, people with kidney disease or epilepsy. Nutritional deficiencies may occur. The one exception is where people choose to fast for religious purposes for which clear health and safety guidelines are provided.

### Bibliography

Jiménez J P, Serrano J, Tabernero M et al 2008 Effects of grape antioxidant dietary fiber in cardiovascular disease risk factors. Nutrition 24(7–8):646–653

Michalsen A 2007 Nutritional and fasting therapy in complementary medicine. Schweiz Zschr GanzheitsMedizin 19(5):260–268

Michalsen A, Hoffmann B, Moebus S 2005 Incorporation of fasting therapy in an integrative medicine ward: evaluation of outcome, safety and effects on lifestyle adherence in a large prospective cohort study. Journal of Alternative and Complementary Medicine 11(4):601–607

# Feingold diet

## Description

This is a pioneering approach in the management of attention deficient hyperactive disorder (ADHD), which involves eliminating additives from the child's diet, specifically fruits and vegetables high in salicylates certain artificial preservatives, synthetic colourings and flavourings. Stage one of the diet lasts from 4 to 6 weeks when all the suspect additives are eliminated.

In stage two, the foods containing natural salicylates are reintroduced and if there is no reaction, a diet is used which only eliminates chemical additives and preservatives. In general, children under 6 years of age respond within 1 week of commencing the diet; children over 6 years of age may take 2–6 weeks to achieve positive results.

Evidence:    There is some evidence to suggest it has a role in helping children with ADHD.

Safety:    No information regarding safety, precautions or contraindications was found, however, caution should be used to ensure that the child remains appropriately nourished. The diet should only be used under supervision.

### Bibliography

Bateman B, Warner J O, Hutchinson E et al 2004 The effects of a double blind, placebo controlled, artificial food colourings and benzoate preservative challenge on hyperactivity in a general population sample of preschool children. Archives of Disease in Childhood 89(6):506–511

Harding K L, Judah R D, Gant C 2003 Outcome-based comparison of Ritalin versus food-supplement treated children with AD/HD. Alternative Medicine Review 8(3):319–330

### Resources

The Feingold Association: www.feingold.org

## Green lipped mussel extract

*Description*

Green lipped mussel extract is derived from *Perna canaliculata*, a salt water shellfish indigenous to New Zealand and traditionally used as an antiinflammatory agent for arthritis, as it contains a weak prostaglandin inhibitor.

Evidence:    supports its traditional use.

Safety:    No information regarding safety, precautions or contraindications was found.

### Bibliography

Cho S H, Jung Y B, Seong S C et al 2003 Clinical efficacy and safety of Lyprinol, a patented extract from New Zealand green-lipped mussel (Perna Canaliculus) in patients with osteoarthritis of the hip and knee: a multicenter 2-month clinical trial. European Annals of Allergy and Clinical Immunology 35(6):212–216

Gibson S L 2000 The effect of a lipid extract of the New Zealand green-lipped mussel in three cases of arthritis. Journal of Alternative and Complementary Medicine 6(4):351–354

Halpern G M 2000 Anti-inflammatory effects of a stabilized lipid extract of Perna canaliculus (Lyprinol). Allergie et immunologie (Paris) 32(7):272–278

Lawson B R, Belkowski S M, Whitesides J F et al 2007 Immunomodulation of murine collagen-induced arthritis by N,N-dimethylglycine and a preparation of Perna canaliculus. BMC Complementary and Alternative Medicine 7:20

Treschow A P, Hodges L D, Wright P F et al 2007 Novel antiinflammatory omega-3 PUFAs from the New Zealand green-lipped mussel, Perna canaliculus. Comparative Biochemistry and Physiology. Part B Biochemistry and Molecular Biology 47(4): 645–656

## Kousmine diet

This is a dietary therapy devised by Dr Catherine Kousmine who claims that multiple sclerosis is caused by poor diet and is curable by following this regimen, involving a low fat, low concentrated sugar, high fibre diet with added vitamins A, C, D, E and B complex. It is recommended that the diet starts with a raw fruit fast followed by 2–3 months avoiding meat.

Evidence:   No specific evidence was found.

Safety:   No information regarding safety and no evidence of contraindications was found. However, it should not be used in place of orthodox medical treatment.

### Bibliography

No professional literature was found.

## Living/raw food diet

*Description*

This is a dietary regimen based on the theory that cooking destroys many of the necessary vitamins and enzymes in food. Some 75% of all food is eaten raw, i.e. uncooked, unheated, unprocessed and organic and consists primarily of wheatgrass juice, fresh and fermented vegetables and fruits and a variety of seeds, nuts, grain, legume and purified water. Milk is taken occasionally but can be made from rice which may then be made into cheese.

The various subgroups include fruitarians who consume mostly fruits, sproutarians who consume mostly sprouts and juicearians who consume mostly fresh juice. It is generally considered a way of life rather than a specific therapeutic intervention.

Evidence:   No evidence of effectiveness for any specific conditions could be found.

Safety:   The diet is very restrictive so it is unsuitable for children, pregnant and lactating women, the elderly and patients with eating disorders. Nutritional deficiencies may occur. Serious weight loss, amenorrhea and low bone mass have been recorded.

### Bibliography

Cunningham E 2004 What is a raw foods diet and are there any risks or benefits associated with it? Journal of the American Dietetic Association 104(10):1623

Fontana L, Shew J L, Holloszy J O et al 2005 Low bone mass in subjects on a long-term raw vegetarian diet. Archives Internal Medicine 165(6):684–689

Gass C, Schlechtriemen M, Klimek J 1999 Dental erosions in subjects living on a raw food diet. Caries Research 33(1):74–80

Hobbs S H 2005 Attitudes, practices and beliefs of individuals consuming a raw foods diet. Explore (NY) 1(4):272–277

Koebnick C, Garcia A L, Dagnelie P C et al 2005 Long-term consumption of a raw food diet is associated with favorable serum LDL cholesterol and triglycerides but also with elevated Plasma homocysteine and low serum HDL cholesterol in humans. Journal of Nutrition 135(10):2372–2378

Koebnick C, Strassner C, Hoffmann I 1999 Consequences of long term raw food diet on body weight and menstruation. Annals of Nutrition and Metabolism 43(2):69–79

## Lorenzo's oil

*Description*

This is a controversial treatment for adrenoleukodystrophy developed by the parents of Lorenzo Odone who was diagnosed with the genetic condition in 1984. Boys carrying the defect have extremely high levels of very long chain saturated fatty acids in their blood and the purpose of the oil, which contains 20% erucic acid and 80% oleic acid, is to attempt to reduce these to normal. Children who have the condition, which affects 16 000 American boys between the ages of 4–10 each year, suffer neurological damage, leading rapidly to paralysis and early death.

Evidence:   Recent research from Johns Hopkins University and the Myelin Project supports the use of the oil in boys identified as carrying the defective gene and before symptoms appear. It has also shown to be of value in other neurological conditions.

Safety: No information regarding safety, and no evidence of contraindications was found.

Bibliography

Ferri R, Chance P F 2005 Lorenzo's oil: advances in the treatment of neurometabolic disorders. Archives of Neurology 62(7):1045–1046

Moser H W, Raymond G V, Koehler W et al 2003 Evaluation of the preventive effect of glyceryl trioleate-trierucate ('Lorenzo's oil') therapy in X-linked adrenoleukodystrophy: results of two concurrent trials. Advances in Experimental Medical Biology 544:369–387

Moser H W, Raymond G V, Lu S E et al 2005 Follow-up of 89 asymptomatic patients with adrenoleukodystrophy treated with Lorenzo's oil. Archives of Neurology 62(7):1073–1080

Moser H W 1999 Treatment of X-linked adrenoleukodystrophy with Lorenzo's oil. Journal of Neurology, Neurosurgery, and Psychiatry 67(3):279–280

Tanaka K, Shimizu T, Ohtsuka Y et al 2007 Early dietary treatments with Lorenzo's oil and docosahexaenoic acid for neurological development in a case with Zellweger syndrome. Brain Development 29(9):586–589

# Macrobiotic diet

*Description*

The macrobiotic dietary regimen was developed by Kushi Ohsawa who claimed to have cured his tuberculosis using this method. It originally consisted of a largely vegetarian diet relying heavily on whole grains and originally had 10 stages, each becoming increasingly restrictive.

Evidence: It is suggested that the macrobiotic diet may have a role in the management of women with breast cancer.

Safety: The diet is very restrictive, not suitable for children, pregnant and lactating women or the elderly. There have been reports of health-related problems due to nutritional deficiencies, specifically vitamin D, B12, iron and calcium. Osteoporosis may be a risk factor and deaths have occurred as a result of the diet.

Bibliography

Berrino F, Villarini A, De Petris M et al 2006 Adjuvant diet to improve hormonal and metabolic factors affecting breast cancer prognosis. Annals of the New York Academy of Science 1089:110–118

Cunningham E, Marcason W 2001 Is there any research to prove that a macrobiotic diet can prevent or cure cancer? Journal of the American Diet Association 101(9):1030

Dhonukshe-Rutten R, van Dusseldorp M, Schneede J et al 2005 Low bone mineral density and bone mineral content are associated with low cobalamin status in adolescents. European Journal of Nutrition 44(6):341–347

Kushi L, Cunningham J, Herbert J et al 2001 The macrobiotic diet in cancer. Journal of Nutrition 131(Suppl):3056S–3064S

Louwman M, van Dusseldorp M, van de Vijver F et al 2000 Signs of impaired cognitive function with adolescents with marginal cobalamin status. American Journal of Clinical Nutrition 72(3):762–769

Parsons T J, van Dusseldorp M, Seibel M J et al 2001 Are levels of bone turnover related to lower bone mass of adolescents previously fed a macrobiotic diet? Experimental and Clinical Endocrinology and Diabetes 109(5):288–293

## Nutraceuticals

*Description*

The term 'nutraceuticals' was coined in 1989 by Stephen De Felice of the American Foundation for the Innovation of Medicine and defined as 'food or part of a food that provides medical or health benefits, including the treatment and prevention of disease'. These cover a range of supplements including herbs, vitamins and minerals, bio-yoghurts (see Probiotics), functional foods, fish oils and fortified cereals. Fish oils contain essential fatty acids and include omega 6 (derived from linoleic acid in vegetables and red meat) and omega 3 (derived from α-linoleic acid in marine plankton and in the flesh of some animals). They are also found in some nuts and oils, i.e. fish and walnut oil. The main types of omega 3 fatty acids are eicosapentanoic acid (EPA) and docosahexanoic acid (DHA), which are now often added to margarine, milk and bread to make them functional foods.

Evidence:   Suggests that omega 3 reduces blood triglyceride levels and also helps to prevent thrombosis and is antiinflammatory. Omega 3's antiinflammatory, anti-thrombolytic properties are used in secondary prevention of coronary heart disease. Omega 6 appears to lower cholesterol but may also lower (HDL) 'good' cholesterol.

Safety:   May enhance triglyceride lowering drugs but can aggravate an increased cholesterol. Caution with blood sugar control in diabetics. Avoid in those on anticoagulants. Some supplements may be contaminated. The Food Advisory Agency advises that children be given supplements only under supervision. Pregnant women should avoid omega 3–6 obtained from fish oils, to avoid excessive vitamin A levels. Dosage should not exceed 3 g daily.

Bibliography

Hadj A, Esmore D, Rowland M 2006 Pre-operative preparation for cardiac surgery utilising a combination of metabolic, physical and mental therapy. Heart, Lung and Circulation 15(3):172–181

Kidd P 2007 Omega 3 DHA and EPA for cognition, behaviour and mood: clinical findings and structural-functional synergies with cell membrane phospholipids. Alternative Medicine Review 12(3):207–227

Lecerf J 2007 Fish products and omega 3 fatty acids: role in preventing cardiovascular disease. Phytotherapie 5(3):HS14–HS21

Mickleborough T, Ionescu A, Rundell K 2004 Omega 3 fatty acids and airway hyper responsiveness in asthma. Journal of Alternative and Complementary Medicine 10(6):1067–1075

Murphy D 2006 Pain. Omega-3 fatty acids (fish oil) as an antiinflammatory: an alternative to non steroidal antiinflammatory drugs for discogenic pain. American Chiropractor 28(9):64–65

Nair G M, Connolly S J 2008 Should patients with cardiovascular disease take fish oil? Canadian Medical Association Journal 178(2):181–182

Sears B 2006 Omega 3 fish oils and diet help ease depression. American Chiropractor 28(13):50–51

Semmes B 2005 Depression: a role for Omega 3 fish oils and B vitamins? Evidence Based Integrated Medicine 2(4):229–237

Surette M E 2008 The science behind dietary omega-3 fatty acids. Canadian Medical Association Journal 178(2):177–180

## Orthomolecular medicine/megavitamin therapy

*Description*

This therapeutic approach involves the medicinal use of large doses of vitamins, minerals and amino acids to counter specific diseases. Linus Pauling claimed that large doses of vitamin C could help cure cancer and studies have indicated that it can enhance the effect of conventional treatments. Diagnosis follows similar lines to conventional medicine with the possibility of additional laboratory tests to determine the patient's nutritional status; may be given alongside or instead of conventional treatment and includes selected nutritional supplements.

Evidence: There is some evidence to suggest that this approach can be helpful in ageing-related disorders, including diabetes, cardiovascular disease, hypertension, age-related deterioration of brain function, vision and immune function.

Safety: Orthodox medication may need to be adjusted if large doses of nutritional supplements are given.

### Bibliography

Janson M 2006 Orthomolecular medicine: the therapeutic use of dietary supplements for anti-aging. Clinical Interventions in Aging 1(3):261–265

Levine S, Saltzman A 2004 Pyridoxine (vitamin B6) neurotoxicity: enhancement by protein-deficient diet. Journal of Applied Toxicology 24(6):497–500

## Probiotics/prebiotics

*Description*

Pro- and prebiotics are nutritional supplements consisting of live microbial food, usually lactobacilli and bifidobacteria cultivated from fermented milk products and taken to improve intestinal microbial balance. Prebiotics are non-digestible food ingredients which stimulate production or increased growth of one or a limited number of commensal colon bacteria.

They have been traditionally used to treat diarrhoea, vaginal infections and raised cholesterol.

Evidence: Clinical trials indicate *Lactobacillus GG* and *Lactobacillus acidophilus* and *Bifidobacteria bifidum* may be useful for travellers' diarrhoea. *Lactobacillus GG* and *enterococcus SF68 Lactobacillus acidophilus, Bifidobacteria longum* and *Lactobacillus casei GG* are indicated for antibiotic-induced and infantile diarrhoea, *Lactobacillus GG* being particularly effective against rotovirus, although this and other probiotics have been shown to be less effective against other organisms. *Lactobacillus acidophilus* in both live and pasteurized yoghurt has a role in preventing vaginal infections, *Lactobacillus GG* and *Bifidobacterium* may assist in preventing and treating eczema. Probiotics have been shown to reduce lactose intolerance and improve lactose digestion. A prebiotic fructo-oligosaccharide with *Lactobacillus acidophilus* or the prebiotic inulin may reduce serum cholesterol.

Safety: Over-the-counter products contain a range of probiotics not all of which may be appropriate for the patient's condition. No specific information regarding safety, contraindications and precautions was found.

### Bibliography

Boyle R, Tang M 2006 The role of probiotics in the management of allergic disease. Clinical Experimental Allergy 36(5):565–568

Dendukuri N, Costa V, McGregor M et al 2005 Probiotic therapy for the prevention and treatment of Clostridium difficile associated diarrhoea: a systematic review. Canadian Medical Association Journal 173(2):167–170

Giovannini M, Agostoni C, Riva E et al 2007 A randomized prospective double blind controlled trial on effects of long term consumption of fermented milk containing Lactobacillus casei in pre school children with allergic asthma and/or rhinitis. Pediatric Research 62(2):215

Grüber C, Wendt M, Sulser C et al 2007 Randomized placebo controlled trial of Lactobacillus rhamnosus GG as treatment for atopic dermatitis in infancy. Allergy 62(11):1270–1276

Lee J, Seto D, Bielory L 2008 Meta-analysis of clinical trials of probiotics for prevention and treatment of pediatric atopic dermatitis. Journal of Allergy Clinical Immunology 121(1):116–121. e11

Niers L, Hoekstra M, Timmerman H et al 2007 Selection of probiotic bacteria for prevention of allergic diseases: immunomodulation of neonatal dendritic cells. Clinical Experimental Immunology 149(2):344–352

Roessler A, Friedrich U, Vogelsang H et al 2008 The immune system in healthy adults and children with atopic dermatitis seems to be affected differently by a probiotic intervention. Clinical Experimental Allergy 38(1):93–102

Vendt N, Grünberg H, Tuure T et al 2006 Growth during the first 6 months of life in infants using formula enriched with Lactobacillus rhamnosus GG: double blind, randomised, controlled trial. Journal of Human Nutrition Dietetics 19(1):51–58

Viljanen M, Savilahti E, Haahtela T 2005 Probiotics in the treatment of atopic eczema/dermatitis syndrome in infants: double blind, placebo controlled trial Allergy 60(4):494–500

# Wheat grass juice

*Description*

Wheat grass juice is a nutritional supplement containing vitamins, A, B, C and K and the minerals, calcium, magnesium, phosphorus, manganese, chlorophyll, potassium, zinc and selenium.

Evidence:    There is clinical evidence of the antiinflammatory effects of wheat grass juice and a possible benefit in gastrointestinal and other conditions.

Safety:    The vitamin K content may interfere with anticoagulant medication.

Bibliography

Bar-Sela G, Tsalic M, Fried G et al 2007 Wheat grass juice may improve haematological toxicity related to chemotherapy in breast cancer patients: a pilot study. Nutrition and Cancer 58(1):43–48

Ben-Ayre E, Goldin E, Wengrower D et al 2002 Wheat grass juice in the treatment of active distal ulcerative colitis: a randomised double-blind placebo controlled trial. Scandinavian Journal of Gastroenterology 37:444–449

Langmead L, Rampton D 2006 Complementary and alternative therapies for inflammatory bowel disease. Alimentary Pharmacology and Therapeutics 23(3):341–349

Marwaha R 2004 Wheat grass juice reduces transfusion requirements in patients with thalassemia major: a pilot study. Indian Pediatrics 41:716–720

Shah S 2007 Dietary factors in the modulation of inflammatory bowel disease activity. Medscape General Medicine 9(1):60

Shyam R, Singh S, Vats P 2007 Wheat grass supplementation decreases oxidative stress in health subjects: comparison study with spirulina. Journal of Alternative and Complementary Medicine 13(8):789–791

Young M, Cook J, Webster K 2006 The effect of topical wheat grass cream on chronic plantar fasciitis: a randomised double-blind placebo controlled trial. Complementary Therapies in Medicine 14(1):3–9

## Art therapy/art psychotherapy/analytical art psychotherapy

*Description*

Art therapy is a form of psychotherapy using the medium of art to enable patients to project their thoughts, feelings and subconscious concerns relating to their illness, to enhance self awareness. It is particularly relevant to people who have suffered sexual or physical abuse or those whose communication skills are impaired. Techniques may include working in papier mache, puppetry, computer-generated graphics and videotaping. Analytical art psychotherapy uses images and archetype in the Jungian manner to facilitate therapy (see also the Anthroposophical medicine section).

Evidence:   Art-based therapies have been shown to aid healing and enhance well-being in a variety of clinical disorders.

Safety:   Therapy should only be undertaken by a skilled therapist with clear referral strategies in place, as appropriate.

Bibliography

Eaton L, Doherty K, Widrick R 2007 A review of research and methods use to establish art therapy as an effective treatment method for traumatised children. Arts in Psychotherapy 34(3):256–262

Feen-Calligan H 2007 The use of art therapy in detoxification from chemical addiction. Canadian Art Therapy Association Journal 20(1):2–15

Freiherr-von-Hornstein W, Gruber H 2006 Art therapy and symptom control: a team approach. European Journal of Palliative Care 13(3):124–126

Gussak D 2006 Effects of art therapy with prison inmates: a follow up study. Arts in Psychotherapy 33(3):188–198

Joseph C 2006 Creative alliance: the healing power of art therapy. Art Therapy 23(1):30–33

Lloyd C, Petchkovsky Wong S 2007 Art and recovery in mental health: a qualitative investigation. British Journal of Occupational Therapy 70(5):207–214

McElroy S, Warren A 2006 Home-based art therapy for older adults with mental health needs: view of clients and caregivers. Art Therapy 23(2):52–58

Orr P 2007 Art therapy with children after disaster: a content analysis. Arts in Psychotherapy 34(4):350–361

Reynolds F, Prior S 2006 The role of art making in identity maintenance: case studies of people living with cancer. European Journal of Cancer Care 15(4):33–41

Smeijsters H, Cleven G 2006 The treatment of aggression using art therapies in forensic psychiatry: results of a qualitative inquiry. Arts in Psychotherapy 33(10):37–58

Tobin B 2006 Art therapy meets EMDR: processing the paper based image with eye movement. Canadian Art Therapy Association Journal 19(2):27–38

Wood M 2007 The benefits of artistic expression in healing. Practice Nurse 18(5):228–234

### Resources

British Association of Art Therapists: www.baat.org

## Bates' method

*Description*

The Bates' method is a system of eyesight training and re-education, developed by William Bates (1860–1931), which attributes defective vision to muscle strain and eschews the use of lenses or surgery as an intervention. Bates' theory was that poor vision was due to tension and strain resulting in misuse of the eyes which, in turn, isolates the person from the environment. It is an educational method in which the student is shown how to relax the eyes, the body and then the eyes and the body together. Treatment involves several exercises to be practised daily, including: palming, cupping the hands over the eyes and inducing relaxation; shifting, looking at a distant object from a different angle and swinging, fixing the eye on a distant object and swinging the head from side-to-side, while keeping the eyes fixed on the target.

Evidence:  No professional clinical research can be found.

Safety:  No information regarding safety and no evidence of contraindications was found. However, caution should be used regarding discarding the use of visual aids for driving, etc.

### Bibliography

No professional literature was found on Bates' eyesight training.

### Resources

Bates' Association for Vision Education: www.seeing.org

## Callahan technique/thought field therapy

*Description*

This unique form of meridian therapy is a natural, non-invasive, drug-free and chemical-free system to rectify and dispel negative or troubled emotions and involves stimulation of meridian points used in applied kinesiology to address the underlying emotional problem. Using these principles, a diagnostic system was devised to identify problems, referred to as perturbations, within the thought field and the development of treatment sequences to address most psychological problems. Germane to this is the use of psychological reversal which is a state or condition, often referred to as psychological block, which inhibits the effectiveness of treatment interventions. This is addressed by reversing the polarity of the meridian being treated.

Evidence:   Review papers suggest a role for thought field therapy in behavioural medicine, while others have explored the physiological effects of the therapy, but there do not appear to be any clinical studies of safety or effectiveness.

Safety:   No information regarding safety, contraindications or precautions was found.

Bibliography

Callahan R J 2001 Raising and lowering of heart rate variability: some clinical findings of thought field therapy. Journal of Clinical Psychology 57(10): 1175–1186

Kline J P 2001 Heart rate variability does not tap putative efficacy of thought field therapy. Journal of Clinical Psychology 57(10):1187–1192, discussion 1251–1260

Sakai C, Paperny D, Mathews M et al 2001 Thought field therapy clinical applications: utilization in an HMO in behavioral medicine and behavioral health services. Journal of Clinical Psychology 57(10):1215–1227

## Chelation therapy

*Description*

Chelation therapy is a chemical process which aims to remove metal or mineral toxins from the body by binding them to an amino acid, ethylendiaminetetraacetic acid (EDTA). It is an orthodox treatment for lead or cadmium poisoning and the removal of zinc, as well as the treatment of cardiovascular disease, but some complementary practitioners use it as a method of detoxification.

Evidence:   None was found.

Safety:   No information regarding safety and no evidence of contraindications was found.

### Bibliography

No professional references regarding the use of chelation therapy by complementary and alternative practitioners could be found.

## Colonic irrigation

### Description

Colonic irrigation is a therapy which has its modern origins in the 19th century health spas of Europe. The aim of the treatment is internal cleansing and detoxification in order to treat conditions such as allergies and addictions. It involves warm, purified water being introduced into the colon via the rectum; the length of the large intestine is infused with a constant stream of water. Abdominal massage is used to stimulate the release of stored faecal matter and other allegedly harmful bacteria. Sometimes herbs, coffee or enzymes may be added to the water.

Evidence:   There is no evidence that the bowel needs to be flushed clean of bacteria to achieve good health, since the gut has a natural colony of the bacteria necessary to maintain the gut flora and to break down fibre.

Safety:   Some danger of bowel perforation, water toxicity and electrolyte imbalance. Contraindicated in inflammatory bowel disorders, high blood pressure. Caution in those with eating disorders. Contraindicated in pregnancy, children and the elderly.

### Bibliography

Handley D V, Rieger N A, Rodda D J 2004 Rectal perforation from colonic irrigation administered by alternative practitioners. Medical Journal of Australia 181(10):575–576

Norlela S, Izham C, Khalid B A 2004 Colonic irrigation-induced hyponatremia. Malaysian Journal of Pathology 26(2):117–118

Richards D G, McMillin D L, Mein E A et al 2006 Colonic irrigations: a review of the historical controversy and the potential for adverse effects. Journal of Alternative and Complementary Medicine 12(4):389–393

Taffinder N J, Tan E, Webb I G et al 2004 Retrograde commercial colonic hydrotherapy. Colorectal Diseases 6(4):258–260

## Dance/drama therapy

*Description*

Dance and drama offer a therapeutic medium for expression and facilitate well-being of the mind–body relationship by improving mood and well-being by raising endorphin levels. It may also be used as reminiscence therapy to reawaken old memories and feelings. It is employed for people with emotional, cognitive, social or physical problems. It enables expression, increased flexibility, vitality and self esteem and provides a vehicle for socialization.

Evidence: There is a reasonable body of evidence to support the use of both dance and drama therapy in various psycho-emotional and traumatic conditions.

Safety: No specific information on safety, contraindications and precautions was found. Therapy is adjusted to accommodate the physical and emotional limitations of the individual. Emotional abreactions may occur.

---

### Bibliography

Couroucli-Robertson K 2001 Brief drama therapy of immigrant adolescent with a speech impediment. Arts in Psychotherapy 28(5):289–297

Hackney M E, Kantorovich S, Levin R et al 2007 Effects of tango on functional mobility in Parkinson's disease: a preliminary study. Journal of Neurologic Physical Therapy 31(4):173–179

Harris D A 2007 Dance/movement therapy approaches to fostering resilience and recovery among African adolescent torture survivors. Torture 17(2):134–155

Henley-Einion A 2007 The ecstasy of spirit: five rhythms for healing. Practising Midwife 10(3):20, 22–23

Jeong Y J, Hong S C, Lee M S et al 2005 Dance movement therapy improves emotional responses and modulates neurohormones in adolescents with mild depression. International Journal of Neuroscience 115(12):1711–1720

Kron J 2006 Creative art therapies. Journal of Complementary Medicine 5(4):26–35

Lahad M 1999 The use of drama therapy with crisis intervention groups, following mass evacuation. Arts in Psychotherapy 26(1):27–33

Landy R 2006 The future of drama therapy. Arts in Psychotherapy 33(2):135–142

Lundy H, McGuffin P 2005 Using dance/movement therapy to augment the effectiveness of therapeutic holding with children. Journal of Child and Adolescent Psychiatric Nursing 18(3):135–145

Pendzik S 2006 On dramatic reality and is therapeutic function in drama therapy. Arts in Psychotherapy 33(4):271–280

Ravelin T, Kylmä J, Korhonen T 2006 Dance in mental health nursing: a hybrid concept analysis. Issues in Mental Health Nursing 27(3):307–317

Rousseau C, Benoit M, Gauthier M F 2007 Classroom drama therapy program for immigrant and refugee adolescents: a pilot study. Clinical Child Psychology and Psychiatry 12(3):451–465

Sandel S L, Judge J O, Landry N 2005 Dance and movement program improves quality-of-life measures in breast cancer survivors. Cancer Nursing 28(4):301–309

### Resources

Association for Dance Movement Therapy: www.dmtuk.co.uk
British Association of Drama Therapy: www.badth.org.uk

## Eclecticism/eclectic medicine

*Description*

The discipline of eclectic medicine was established in America in the 19th century and utilizes a range of therapeutic interventions, from a variety of medical traditions as appropriate, most commonly, allopathic medicine, homeopathy, naturopathy and herbalism but also including Native American medical theories.

Evidence: There is little research on the overall concept of eclectic medicine, although the individual components have all been investigated widely. There is some suggestion that an eclectic approach to management may be useful in mental illness and learning disability care.

Safety: No specific safety information regarding contraindications and precautions was found. Refer to the safety information for the individual aspects of the therapeutic approach.

### Bibliography

Bodkin J A, Klitzman R L, Pope H G Jr. 1995 Treatment orientation and associated characteristics of North American academic psychiatrists. Journal of Nervous and Mental Disease 183(12):729–735

Brendel D H 2003 Reductionism, eclecticism and pragmatism in psychiatry: the dialectic of clinical explanation. Journal of Medicine and Philosophy 28(5–6):563–580

Kidd P M 2002 Autism, an extreme challenge to integrative medicine. Part 2: medical management. Alternative Medicine Review 7(6):472–499

## Eye movement desensitization and reprocessing (EMDR)

*Description*

EMDR is a technique developed by Francine Shapiro in 1987 used to treat post-traumatic stress disorder. It is based on the theory that humans have a physiologically based information-processing system. When a traumatic or negative event occurs, information-processing may be incomplete, possibly due to disassociation. If information-processing is uninterrupted, memories are stored appropriately, but interference in the processing system causes the memories to be inappropriately stored and to resurface periodically in response to external or internal stimuli. EMDR seeks to reprogramme the processing system to enable memories to be stored appropriately. The exact mechanism is unclear but rapid lateral eye movements as well as other rhythmic tapping or alternating audio tones in the client's ear could help people to reprocess traumatic memories in a less distressing way. It has also been suggested that the EMDR processing system is akin to the rapid eye movements which occur during REM sleep, when dreaming takes place; research indicates that memories are often played out during sleep, processed and stored.

Evidence:   Care reports and randomized controlled trials support the use of the technique in the treatment of post-traumatic stress disorder.

Safety:   The therapy is safe in the hands of a suitably qualified clinical psychologist.

Bibliography

Ahmad A, Larsson B, Sundelin-Wahlsten V 2007 EMDR treatment for children with PTSD: results of a randomized controlled trial. Nordic Journal of Psychiatry 61(5):349–354

Bisson J I, Ehlers A, Matthews R 2007 Psychological treatments for chronic post-traumatic stress disorder. Systematic review and meta-analysis. British Journal of Psychiatry 190:97–104

Keenan P, Royle L 2007 Vicarious trauma and first responders: a case study utilizing eye movement desensitization and reprocessing (EMDR) as the primary treatment modality. International Journal of Emergency Mental Health 9(4):291–298

Lee C W, Drummond P D 2007 Effects of eye movement versus therapist instructions on the processing of distressing memories. Journal of Anxiety Disorders 22(5):801–808

Letizia B, Andrea F, Paolo C 2007 Neuroanatomical changes after eye movement desensitization and reprocessing (EMDR) treatment in posttraumatic stress disorder. Journal of Neuropsychiatry Clinical Neurosciences 19(4): 475–476

Sack M, Lempa W, Steinmetz A 2008 Alterations in autonomic tone during trauma exposure using eye movement desensitization and reprocessing (EMDR): results of a preliminary investigation. Journal of Anxiety Disorders 22(7):1264–1271

Schneider J, Hofmann A, Rost C et al 2008 EMDR in the treatment of chronic phantom limb pain. Pain Medicine 9(1):76–82

## Humour/laughter therapy

*Description*

This interactive therapy was developed by the American physician, Patch Adams and involves the use of humour and laughter, theatre, verbal and physical play to engender feelings of well-being and to aid recovery. The therapy now includes outreach progammes which aim to bring laughter and entertainment to hospitalized patients. For children, a circus-based approach is used involving jugglers, clowns, dancers, etc. And for adults, notably those who are too ill to leave their beds, volunteers devise strategies to set up humorous incidents within the hospital so that patients may interact more positively with the medical and nursing staff. Laughing spirit listening circles involve a group of up to 10 people who each pledge to receive positive attention, initially for 3 min, then for 5 min; as feelings of security grow, participants 'lighten up' and laughter ensues.

Evidence:   It can help to facilitate insight through metaphor, joke or story; the act of laughing has been shown to increase oxygenation of the blood and muscle relaxation.

Safety:   No evidence was found related to safety, contraindications or precautions.

Bibliography

Kissane D W, Grabsch B, Clarke D M et al 2004 Supportive-expressive group therapy: the transformation of existential ambivalence into creative living while enhancing adherence to anti-cancer therapies. Psychooncology 13(11): 755–768

Parslow R, Morgan A J, Allen N B et al 2008 Effectiveness of complementary and self-help treatments for anxiety in children and adolescents. Medical Journal of Australia 188(6):355–359

Phipps S 2002 Reduction of distress associated with paediatric bone marrow transplant: complementary health promotion interventions. Pediatric Rehabilitation 5(4):223–234, Review

Sullivan T, Weinert C, Cudney S 2003 Management of chronic illness: voices of rural women. Journal of Advanced Nursing 44(6):566–574

Walter M, Hänni B, Haug M et al 2007 Humour therapy in patients with late-life depression or Alzheimer's disease: a pilot study. International Journal of Geriatric Psychiatry 22(1):77–83

Walker J A 2002 Emotional and psychological preoperative preparation in adults. British Journal of Nursing 11(8):567–575

Walter M, Hänni B, Haug M et al 2007 Humour therapy in patients with late-life depression or Alzheimer's disease: a pilot study. International Journal of Geriatric Psychiatry 22(1):77–83

# Live cell therapy

*Description*

Live cell therapy is a therapeutic technique originally developed in the 1930s by Dr Paul Niehans, a Swiss endocrinologist, although the original concept is said to be recorded in ancient documents. It involves the injection of living cells, obtained from embryos or animal organs, to correct a range of conditions. Most commonly used were cell extracts from pituitary or adrenal glands, the ovaries, testes and other organs. The theory purported that new live cells would replace damaged or worn cells and improve organ functioning. Products currently available do not contain live cells, but protein extracts from living cells, which have been purified and preserved.

Evidence:   No specific evidence was found.

Safety:   No information regarding safety or contraindications was found. However, allergic reaction is possible. Not to be used by people with current infection.

Bibliography

Chen H, Ouyang W, Jones M et al 2007 Preparation and characterization of novel polymeric microcapsules for live cell encapsulation and therapy. Cell Biochemistry and Biophysics 47(1):159–168

## Music therapy

*Description*

Music can be used therapeutically to enable people to express their emotions and feelings about their illness and is particularly helpful for people with impaired communication and for children. It provides psychological comfort and can be used as part of reminiscence therapy. Techniques may include encouraging patients to write songs or play an instrument. Anthroposophical medicine uses music therapy as an integral part of the diagnostic and healing process.

Evidence:    Physical variations measured during music therapy include changes in metabolism, heart rate, blood pressure and energy levels.

Safety:    No specific evidence regarding safety, contraindications or precautions could be found. Healthcare professionals should be alert to the emotional effects of music and have referral strategies in place as necessary.

Bibliography

Amadoru S, McFerran K 2007 The role of music therapy in children's hospices. European Journal of Palliative Care 14(3):124–127

Baker F, Gleadhill L, Thy M et al 2007 Music therapy and emotional exploration: exposing substance abuse clients to the experiences of non-drug induced emotions. Arts in Psychotherapy 34(4):321–330

Bodner E, Iancu J, Gilboa A et al 2007 finding words for emotions: the reactions of patients with major depressive disorder towards various musical excerpts. Arts in Psychotherapy 34(2):142–150

Boso M, Emanuele E, Minazzi V et al 2007 Effect of long term interactive music therapy on behavior profile and musical skills in young adults with severe autism. Journal of Alternative and Complementary Medicine 13(7):709–712

Cobbett S 2007 Combining music therapy with other creative therapies in individual work with children with emotional and behavioural difficulties. British Journal of Music Therapy 21(1):3–11

Dingle G A, Gleadhill L, Baker F A 2008 Can music therapy engage patients in group cognitive behaviour therapy for substance abuse treatment? Drug and Alcohol Review 27(2):190–196

Groen K 2007 Pain assessment and management in end of life care: a survey of assessment and treatment practices of hospice music therapy and nursing professionals. Journal of Music Therapy 44(2):90–112

Hendon C, Bohon L M 2008 Hospitalized children's mood differences during play and music therapy. Child Care Health Disease 34(2):141–144

Podder L 2007 Effects of music therapy on anxiety levels and pain perception. Nursing Journal of India 98(7):161

Suda M, Morimoto K, Obata A et al 2008 Emotional responses to music: towards scientific perspectives on music therapy. Neuroreport 19(1):75–78

## Resources

Association of Professional Music Therapists: www.apmt.org.uk
British Society for Music Therapy: www.bsmt.org.uk

# R

## Relaxation therapies

*Definition*

Relaxation is a generic term covering a range of techniques which release physical and mental tension from the body and are useful for people with conditions in which stress and anxiety are precipitating or exacerbating factors.

There are many different forms of relaxation training and therapy. Release-only methods include cue-controlled relaxation, which teaches relaxation cued with a trigger word, until the word itself induces a feeling of relaxation; Madders relaxation works by instructing the patient to focus on different parts of the body and note any tension felt, relaxation being achieved by consciously 'letting go'; the Kermani scanning technique involves mentally scanning the body to identify muscular tension which is relieved through passive muscular relaxation. Passive muscular relaxation is accomplished through a systematic review of muscle groups and identification of any tension which is subsequently released, using relaxation through recall, passive neuromuscular relaxation, Kermani's scanning technique and a relaxation ripple. A relaxation ripple consists of one continuous wave of relaxation, timed to coincide with exhalation, starting at the head and sweeping down through the body to the toes, releasing tension where it is identified.

Deep relaxation uses a quiet environment with the person lying supine and involves a process of total body relaxation resulting in a profoundly relaxing effect; conversely, brief relaxation, derived from progressive relaxation and autogenic training, allows the person to achieve an immediate state of relaxation when faced with a stressful situation; while rapid relaxation uses environmental objects as cues to induce relaxation such as a wrist-watch or telephone. Differential relaxation concentrates on controlling muscle tension and teaching the person to become aware of tension levels within various muscle groups and may be used in conjunction with cue-controlled relaxation. Electro-dermal response biofeedback uses sensors to monitor and feedback skin conductance in order to treat anxiety disorders, chronic pain and stress. Behavioural relaxation training is an aspect of cognitive behavioural therapy in which the client self-induces relaxation by assuming the appearance of being relaxed (whatever their feelings), thus inducing genuine feelings of relaxation. Brainwave training/neurofeedback teaches patients to identify, control and enhance brainwave activity in order to treat addictions, seizures and sleep disorders. The Mitchell method is based on the principle of reciprocal inhibition, i.e. when one group of muscles is working, the opposite group of muscles is relaxed; it aims to reduce stress and relax the mind by recognizing the difference between muscular tension and relaxation, combined with visualization and a breathing technique in which the person is encouraged to 'sigh out slowly', focussing on expiration, rather than inhalation.

Evidence:   There is evidence of the physiological benefits of different forms of relaxation and their uses in a variety of clinical conditions, including hypertension, headaches and other sources of pain, anxiety, stress and other psychological disorders.

Safety:   Relaxation training is contraindicated in acute psychotic states or those susceptible to psychosis but may benefit the patient during a non-active period of illness; trance-like states can lead to feelings of disorientation and depersonalization and should not be entered into for long periods of time. Emotional abreaction may occur.

### Bibliography

Butnik S M 2005 Neurofeedback in adolescents and adults with attention deficit hyperactivity disorder. Journal of Clinical Psychology 61(5):621–625

Huntley A, White A, Ernst E 2002 Relaxation therapies for asthma: a systematic review. Thorax 57(2):127–131

Jensen M P, Hakimian S, Sherlin L H et al 2008 New insights into neuromodulatory approaches for the treatment of pain. Journal of Pain 9(3):193–199

Joshi S 2008 Nonpharmacologic therapy for insomnia in the elderly. Clinics in Geriatric Medicine 24(1):107–119, viii

Kuijpers H J, van der Heijden F M, Tuinier S et al 2007 Meditation-induced psychosis. Psychopathology 40(6):461–464

Lahmann C, Schoen R, Henningsen P et al 2008 Brief relaxation versus music distraction in the treatment of dental anxiety: a randomized controlled clinical trial. Journal of the American Dental Association 139(3):317–324

Lovas J G, Lovas D A 2007 Rapid relaxation: practical management of preoperative anxiety. Journal of the Canadian Dental Association 73(5):437–440

Smitherman T A, Penzien D B, Rains J C 2007 Challenges of nonpharmacologic interventions in chronic tension-type headache. Current Pain and Headache Reports 11(6):471–477

van der Veek P P, van Rood Y R, Masclee A A 2007 Clinical trial: short- and long-term benefit of relaxation training for irritable bowel syndrome. Alimentary Pharmacology and Therapeutics 26(6):943–952

Wardell D, Rintala D, Duan Z et al 2006 A pilot study of healing touch and progressive relaxation for chronic neuropathic pain with spinal chord injury. Journal of Holistic Nursing 24(4):231–240.

## Autogenic training

### Description

Autogenic training encourages an altered form of consciousness, while the brain and physical body function normally, facilitating homeostasis. It is based on the philosophy of empowering the person to continue therapy without the trainer being present. It can induce deep relaxation, reducing stress and aiding pain management and has been used to treat migraine, hypertension, asthma, digestive problems, eczema and anxiety.

Evidence:    Case reports and some formal trials indicate a use for autogenic training in the management of pain and stress.

Safety:    No specific safety issues were found.

### Bibliography

Goto F, Nakai K, Kunihiro T et al 2008 Case report: a case of intractable Meniere's disease treated with autogenic training. Biopsychosocial Medicine 2:3

Ishikawa K, Saito M 2008 Self-care for job stress in the workplace. Sangyo Eiseigaku Zasshi 50(1):4–10

Kanji N 2000 Management of pain through autogenic training. Complementary Therapies in Nursing and Midwifery 6(3):143–148

Kanji N, Ernst E 2000 Autogenic training for stress and anxiety: a systematic review. Complementary Therapies in Medicine 8:106–110

Stetter F, Kupper S 2002 Autogenic training: a meta-analysis of clinical outcome studies. Applied Psychophysiology and Biofeedback 27(1):45–98

Sugimoto K, Theoharides T C, Kempuraj D et al 2007 Response of spinal myoclonus to a combination therapy of autogenic training and biofeedback. Biopsychosocial Medicine 1:18

Weisser B 2007 Relaxation techniques for patients with high blood pressure. MMW Fortschritte der Medizin 149(45):45–46

Resources

British Autogenic Society: www.autogenic-therapy.org.uk

# Biofeedback

*Description*

Biofeedback involves educating clients about body movements by using monitors or computer-aided graphical instrumentation to monitor, amplify and feedback physiological information to enable them to exert conscious control over autonomic functions. It works on the principle inherent in any learning – that information or knowledge about results is necessary to acquire a skill; in this case, greater control over a biological function such as heart rate or blood pressure. Biofeedback instruments include monitors to measure skin resistance, skin temperature, muscle activity and electroencephalograph monitors.

Evidence:   Biofeedback has been used successfully to treat problems in which voluntary muscular control is deficient, e.g. pelvic floor and respiratory muscles; it has also been used in the treatment of stress-related skin conditions and for substance dependence.

Safety:   No specific safety issues were found.

Bibliography

Ansari M S, Srivastava A, Kapoor R et al 2008 Biofeedback therapy and home pelvic floor exercises for lower urinary tract dysfunction after posterior urethral valve ablation. Journal of Urology 179(2):708–711

Conde Pastor M, Javier Menéndez F, Sanz M T et al 2008 The influence of respiration on biofeedback techniques. Applied Psychophysiology and Biofeedback 33(1):49–54

Fried R G, Hussain S H 2008 Nonpharmacologic management of common skin and psycho-cutaneous disorders. Dermatologic Therapy 21(1):60–68

Lourenção M I, Battistella L R, de Brito C M et al 2008 Effect of biofeedback accompanying occupational therapy and functional electrical stimulation in hemiplegic patients. International Journal of Rehabilitation Research 31(1):33–41

Reiner R 2008 Integrating a portable biofeedback device into clinical practice for patients with anxiety disorders: results of a pilot study. Applied Psychophysiology Biofeedback 33(1):55–61

Sokhadze T M, Cannon R L, Trudeau D L 2008 EEG biofeedback as a treatment for substance use disorders: review, rating of efficacy and recommendations for further research. Applied Psychophysiology Biofeedback 33(1):1–28

Resources

Biofeedback Foundation of Europe: www.bfe.org

## Floatation therapy

*Description*

Floatation therapy is thought to induce deep relaxation via severely reduced sensory input. The person floats in a solution of salt water, warmed to blood heat, in near or complete darkness and in complete silence or with music or nature sounds if preferred, so that the brain releases endorphins, leading to pain relief and feelings of euphoria.

Evidence:    There is some emerging evidence to support its use in treating muscle pain.

Safety:    Care should be taken when used by people who are prone to claustrophobia.

Bibliography

Bood S A, Sundequist U, Kjellgren A 2005 Effects of flotation-restricted environmental stimulation technique on stress-related muscle pain: what makes the difference in therapy – attention-placebo or the relaxation response? Pain Research Management 10(4):201–209

Hu P C, Su Y 2004 Effects of flotation therapy on relaxation and mental state. Chinese Medicine Journal (Engl) 117(10):1579–1581

Kjellgren A, Sundequist U, Norlander T 2001 Effects of flotation-REST on muscle tension pain. Pain Research Management 6(4):181–189

Resources

Floatation Tank Association: www.floatationtankassociation.net

## Jacobson's progressive relaxation

*Description*

This technique is based on the theory that thinking is related to muscle state, thus muscle relaxation produces a calm and peaceful state of mind, calming the whole person, leading to greater clarity of thought and a greater facility to think through and solve emotional problems. Full training takes approximately 50 sessions, as only two new muscle groups are introduced at each session.

Evidence: Evidence supports its role in reducing stress, anxiety and insomnia and is of benefit in conditions where stress and anxiety are a predisposing or aggravating factor.

Safety: No specific safety issues were found.

### Bibliography

Greeff A, Conradie W 1998 Use of progressive relaxation training for chronic alcoholics with insomnia. Psychological Reports 82(2):407–412

Salt V, Kerr K 1997 Mitchell's simple physiological relaxation and Jacobson's progressive relaxation techniques: a comparison. Physiotherapy 83(4):200–207

Takaishi N 2000 A comparative study of autogenic training and progressive relaxation as methods for teaching clients to relax. Sleep and Hypnosis 2(3):132–137

# Meditation

*Description*

Meditation employs a range of techniques to relax, facilitate deep reflection and clear the mind. Concentrative meditation encourages the person to concentrate on a sound or word (mantra), colour or personal or religious icon, which is silently repeated over and over again to prevent distracting thought intruding on the mind. If distracting thoughts intrude the person is instructed to be passive and return to the mantra, e.g. Transcendental Meditation™ popularized by the Maharishi Mahesh Yogi, in which the secret mantra is given to each person by the trainer and Benson's Relaxation response, developed from Transcendental Meditation™, which encourages the relaxation response as a state of decreased psycho-physiological arousal, synonymous with parasympathetic activity, by using a mental device similar to a mantra – but any phrase chosen by the patient is used as a focal point of attention to induce mental stillness and a passive attitude. The TM-Sidhi programme is an advanced meditation practice, including yogic flying, which allows a meditator to explore the deeper states of consciousness through regular practice of transcendental meditation. Vedic mantra meditation involves the use of a single sound on which to concentrate, to which no attitudes or emotions are attached.

Mindful meditation encourages the person to be mindful of all surrounding sensations, including feelings, images, thoughts and sound, with the aim of cultivating an intentionally non-reactive, non-judgemental, moment-to-moment awareness. Meditation requires a quiet environment, comfortable position and sometimes a mental tool, such as a mantra. Active meditation employs breathing, movement, visualization and exercises to improve self-awareness.

Evidence:  There is evidence of successful use of meditation for conditions induced by stress, including occupational burnout, skin and anxiety problems.

Safety:  No specific safety issues were found.

### Bibliography

Anderson J W, Liu C, Kryscio R J 2008 Blood pressure response to transcendental meditation: a meta-analysis. American Journal of Hypertension 21(3):310–316

Davies W R 2008 Mindful meditation: healing burnout in critical care nursing. Holistic Nursing Practice 22(1):32–36

Dusek J A, Hibberd P L, Buczynski B et al 2008 Stress management versus lifestyle modification on systolic hypertension and medication elimination: a randomized trial. Journal of Alternative and Complementary Medicine 14(2):129–138

Fried R G, Hussain S H 2008 Nonpharmacologic management of common skin and psychocutaneous disorders. Dermatological Therapies 21(1):60–68

Huynh T V, Gotay C, Layi G et al 2007 Mindfulness meditation and its medical and non-medical applications. Hawaii Medical Journal 66(12):328–330

Kim T S, Park J S, Kim M A 2008 The relation of meditation to power and well-being. Nursing Science Quarterly 21(1):49–58

Swinehart R 2008 Two cases support the benefits of transcendental meditation in epilepsy. Medical Hypotheses 70(5):1070

### Resources

Transcendental Meditation: www.transcendental-meditation.org.uk
Henry-Benson Institute of Mind-Body Medicine: www.mbmi.org

## Snoezelen

*Description*

Snoezelen was developed from the Dutch words meaning 'sniffing' and 'dozing' at the Hartenburg Centre in the Netherlands and focuses on sensory perception. A Snoezelen room consists of pleasurable sensory experiences of light, colour, sound and smell to induce feelings of relaxation and calm. The basic room colour can be black or white, a white room being most suitable for light and colour therapy using bubble tubes and fibreoptics, while a black one is for sound rhythms using a variety of musical pitches, sounds and musical instruments, visual tracking, deep relaxation and concentration. Benefits of this therapy have been noted in a range of conditions including dementia, learning difficulties, autism and physical conditions where stress, pain and anxiety are a factor.

Evidence: supports its use for the treatment of brain injury, relaxation during labour and improves quality of life for the disabled.

Safety: No specific information was found regarding safety, contraindications or precautions.

### Bibliography

Ball J, Haight B K 2005 Creating a multisensory environment for dementia: the goals of a Snoezelen room. Journal of Gerontology Nursing 31(10):4–10

Hauck Y, Rivers C, Doherty K 2007 Women's experiences of using a Snoezelen room during labour in Western Australia. Midwifery 27 Jul [Epub ahead of print]

Hotz G A, Castelblanco A, Lara I M 2006 Snoezelen: a controlled multi-sensory stimulation therapy for children recovering from severe brain injury. Brain Injury 20(8):879–888

Lavie E, Shapiro M, Julius M 2005 Hydrotherapy combined with Snoezelen multi-sensory therapy. International Journal of Adolescent Medical Health 17(1):83–87

Livingston G, Johnston K, Katona C et al 2005 Systematic review of psychological approaches to the management of neuropsychiatric symptoms of dementia. American Journal of Psychiatry 162(11):1996–2021

Lotan M, Shapiro M 2005 Management of young children with Rett disorder in the controlled multi-sensory (Snoezelen) environment. Brain Development 27 (Suppl 1):S88–S94

Rivers C, Doherty K, Hauck Y 2007 Use of the Snoezelen concept for maternity clients. Australian Nursing Journal 15(3):35

van Weert J C, van Dulmen A M, Spreeuwenberg P M et al 2005 Effects of Snoezelen, integrated in 24 h dementia care, on nurse-patient communication during morning care. Patient Education and Counseling 58(3):312–326

# T

## Traditional systems of medicine

*Description*

Indigenous medicine – a generic term referring to the traditional healing practices around the world – uses informal local knowledge and resources, such as herbal and homemade remedies. Shamanism is a spiritual tradition common to many cultures with a history of at least 30 000 years and addresses issues of change and growth, particularly rites of passage, such as birth, marriage, death, etc. Germane to its practice is the Shamanic State of Consciousness enabling the Shaman to access knowledge, insight and wisdom which are otherwise inaccessible. Shamanic healing involves exploring the meaning of the illness to the patient and the exploration of appropriate interventions acceptable to the patient, including drumming, dancing, chanting, dreaming and healing ceremonies.

Indigenous or folk medicine is distinct from scientific knowledge, but may include more formal and systematic, but largely unproven (at least in the west), medical practices such as Indian Ayurvedic, traditional Chinese medicine, Japanese kampo and South African muthi, although there is an increasing body of knowledge regarding specific aspects of traditional medicine, such as research studies on individual herbal remedies. Interventions are culturally determined, affordable and acceptable to the population they serve; healers are trained usually through apprenticeship to a charismatic teacher and the work is entered into by inheritance or through a divine calling. Remedies recognized to have healing properties have usually been accumulated through custom and practice, often over the course of centuries and vary from herbal remedies to over-the-counter preparations, as well as those passed down by word of mouth.

Evidence:   There is little direct evidence of the individual systems of traditional medicine, but several studies have been undertaken on the effectiveness and safety of specific herbal remedies from many areas of the world. The professional literature in English seems to debate the biosocial aspects of traditional medicine use within developed and developing countries, with some covering the potential for herbal interactions with conventional pharmacological preparations and others exploring the cultural diversity and ethical issues inherent in what is essentially 'folk medicine'. Other studies have investigated the specific elements of a particular medical system, such as acupuncture within traditional Chinese medicine, shiatsu in Japanese medicine, the use of various procedures and traditional practices, such as circumcision within African medicine or individual herbs from around the world.

Safety: Issues pertaining to the safety of various components of traditional medicine have been documented, e.g. the risks of acupuncture needles being left in situ; the possibility of burns from moxibustion; the dangers of herb–drug interactions; and concern over delayed treatment with conventional healthcare when traditional medicine is used as the primary source of treatment. There are also case reports of problems such as gangrene from traditional bone setters and hepatitis risk resulting from poor hygiene during traditional procedures.

## Bibliography

Alves R R, Rosa I M 2007 Biodiversity, traditional medicine and public health: where do they meet? Journal of Ethnobiology and Ethnomedicine 3:14

Aginam O 2007 Beyond shamanism: the relevance of African traditional medicine in global health policy. Medicine and Law 26(2):191–201

Cadit A A 2007 Role of shamans in a multidisciplinary mental health team Journal of the College of Physicians and Surgeons – Pakistan 17(3):183–184

Hyman M A 2007 The first mind-body medicine: bringing shamanism into the 21st century. Alternative Therapies in Health and Medicine 13(5):10–11

Nauman E 2007 Native American medicine and cardiovascular disease. Cardiology in Review 15(1):35–41

Omonzejele P F 2008 African concepts of health, disease and treatment: an ethical inquiry. Explore (NY) 4(2):120–126

Peltzer K, Nqeketo A, Petros G et al 2008 Traditional circumcision during manhood initiation rituals in the Eastern Cape, South Africa: a pre-post intervention evaluation. BMC Public Health 8:64

Reihling H C 2008 Bioprospecting the African Renaissance: the new value of muthi in South Africa. Journal of Ethnobiology and Ethnomedicine 4(1):9

Viladrich A 2007 From 'shrinks' to 'urban shamans': Argentine immigrants' therapeutic eclecticism in New York City. Culture, Medicine, and Psychiatry 31(3):307–328

## Resources

World Health Organization: www.who.int/gb/ebwha

## Ayurvedic medicine

*Description*

Ayurveda is a traditional form of Indian medicine, about 5000 years old, the term derived from *ayur* (life) and *veda* (knowledge) and is based on the principle of primordial energy, which is central to health maintenance. It is believed that the universe comprises five elements: air (*prana*), fire, earth, ether/space and water, which are in a state of perpetual motion interacting with each other. Prana is the vital energy thought to activate body and mind, which circulates round the body through a series of energy channels (*nadis*) permeating organs and tissues, especially concentrated at the chakras and responsible for the higher cerebral functions, motor and sensory activities. It is similar in concept to the Qi or Chinese medicine, the Ki in Japanese medicine and the vital force of homeopathy. In combination, the five elements form the three vital *doshas* or energies, known as *Tridosha*, which, together with the seven *dhatus* (vital tissues) and the three *malas* (waste products of sweat, urine and faeces), make up the human body.

There are also three mental states. Tridosha comprises three energies representing physical and psychological aspects of the individual, which make up the constitution. Imbalances between the doshas reduce the body's natural resistance, leaving the person open to illness and disease. People are encouraged to lead their lives in accordance with their predominant dosha. *Kapha* or *phlegm dosha*, a combination of water and earth, is thought to regulate pitta and vata. Kapha is considered to be the cerebral core, responsible for keeping the body lubricated, also for tissues and for strength. Conditions in which kapha is dominant include catarrh, influenza, heart disease, excess weight, diabetes, water retention and digestive conditions. *Pitta* or *bile*, is a combination of fire and water, responsible for digestion and metabolism, courage and mental activity; resides in the middle body, primarily the stomach. Conditions in which pitta predominates include skin rashes, fever, inflammation, eye problems (e.g. conjunctivitis) and gastric upsets. *Vata* or *wind*, is a combination of air and ether, responsible for body movements and nervous energy and resides in the lower body, primarily the colon. When vata dominates individuals, they are likely to suffer from emotional illnesses, nervous system disorders, depression, anxiety, constipation and mental confusion. *Chakras* (wheels) – seven energy centres along the midline of the body – the crown, brow, throat, heart, solar plexus, sacral and base chakras, are responsible for the transmission and reception of energies from the consciousness through the endocrine and nervous systems to other parts of the body via a system of energy channels called *Nadis*. Each chakra has a different form, colour and energy vibration.

Ayurvedic diagnosis uses eight classical methods of examination: *Nadi* (pulse) is the most important aspect of diagnosis, involving palpation of the right radial artery in men and left radial artery in women, at the base of the thumb, with the clinician using three fingers. Pulse presentation depends on the dominant dosha, e.g. a pulse resembling a snake under the index finger indicates predominance of vata, a pulse resembling a frog under the middle finger indicates Pitta and pulse under the ring finger resembling a swan or peacock, a predominance of Kapha. *Jihva* (tongue) – the tongue is regarded as a reflection of the internal organs and its appearance, colour and shape will help to determine which of the tridosha is unbalanced. A whitish tongue indicates a kapha disorder with mucus accumulation; a red or yellow/green tongue indicates pitta disorder; a black or brown discoloration indicates a vata condition. A dehydrated tongue may indicate decreased *Dhatu* (vital tissue) or *Rasa* (plasma); a pale tongue indicates decreased *Dhatu Rakta* (red blood cells). A line down the middle of the tongue indicates that emotions are being held in the spinal column. *Druga* (eyes) – examination of the eyes may indicate imbalances within the tridosha, e.g. Vata eyes are small, blink frequently, may have dry scanty lashes and drooping eyelids, the white of the eye is muddy with a dark iris. Pitta eyes are of moderate size lustrous and sensitive to light, eyelashes are scanty and oily and the iris is red or yellowish. Kapha eyes are large, beautiful and moist with long thick lashes, the white of the eye is clear and the iris is pale blue or black. *Mutra* (urine, see below) is examined to determine dosha predominance, e.g. pale yellow urine indicates Vata; intense yellow, reddish or blue urine indicates Pitta, white foamy, muddy urine indicates Kapha. Other aspects of diagnosis include *Mala* (faeces); *Shabda* (speech and voice); *Sparsha* (physical examination by palpation) and *Akruti*, a general physical examination.

Treatment consists of prophylaxis to maintain good health and therapy to treat ill-health. *Panchakarma* (five action treatment) is a deep cleansing process consisting of a 3-, 7- or 30-day course of treatment. The person is prepared with oil massage and sweat therapy, then treatment may include therapeutic vomiting, purgatives and laxatives, therapeutic enemas, nasal administration of medicines and/or purification of the blood. Treatment may also consist of the use of honey, butter/ ghee or sesame oil to eliminate Kapha, Pitta and Vata, respectively; gem and colour therapy, dietary adjustment to re-balance the doshas, Indian herbal medicines, marma therapy – based on massage of 107 subcutaneous pressure points connecting body and mind, aimed to re-balance the tridosha, promote healing, enhance immunity and raise serotonin levels – as well as Indian head massage and yoga (see below). Indian head massage incorporates massage of the upper back, scalp and face to reduce accumulated tension, stimulate circulation and restore joint movement.

Safety:   Head massage should not be performed on people with acute intracranial haemorrhage or pressure, aneurysm or recent skull fracture.

Evidence:   Ayurvedic medicine has been shown in a few small-scale research studies to have a possible role in the management of people with schizophrenia. Kachnar, an herbal remedy, appears to have a hepato-protective function and *Triphala guggulu* (myrrh) may be chondroprotective. 'Ilogen-Excel', a combination herbal remedy, may be useful in reducing glucose levels in diabetic patients, but conversely may interfere with serum glucose levels in those requiring insulin, while systematic reviews of various studies suggest that other Ayurvedic combination remedies may reduce hyperlipidaemia.

Safety:   Certain herbal remedies may interfere with conventional pharmacology, including Ashwagandha, which has a similar structure to digoxin and may interfere with serum digoxin measurements in cardiac patients.

Bibliography

Agarwal V, Abhijnhan A, Raviraj P 2007 Ayurvedic medicine for schizophrenia. Cochrane Database of Systematic Reviews(4): CD006867

Dasgupta A, Peterson A, Wells A et al 2007 Effect of Indian Ayurvedic medicine Ashwagandha on measurement of serum digoxin and 11 commonly monitored drugs using immunoassays: study of protein binding and interaction with Digibind. Archives of Pathology and Laboratory Medicine 131(8):1298–1303

Elder C 2004 Ayurveda for diabetes mellitus: a review of the biomedical literature. Alternative Therapies in Health and Medicine 10(1):44–50

Elder C, Aickin M, Bauer V et al 2006 Randomised trial of a whole system Ayurvedic protocol for type 2 diabetes. Alternative Therapies in Health and Medicine 12(5):24–30

Jagtap A, Shirke S, Phadke A 2004 Effect of polyherb formulation on experimental models of inflammatory bowel disease. Journal of Ethnopharmacology 90(2–3): 195–204

Singh B B, Vinjamury S P, Der-Martirosian C et al 2007 Ayurvedic and collateral herbal treatments for hyperlipidemia: a systematic review of randomized controlled trials and quasi-experimental designs. Alternative Therapies in Health and Medicine 13(4):22–28

Sumantran V N, Kulkarni A A, Harsulkar A et al 2007 Hyaluronidase and collagenase inhibitory activities of the herbal formulation Triphala guggulu. Journal of Bioscience 32(4):755–761

Resources

Ayurvedic Medical Association UK: www.ayurvedicmedicalassociation.com

## Yoga

Yoga – or union – involves postures (*asanas*), breathing exercises (*pranayama*) and meditation (*dhyana*), practised in various proportional mixes depending on the predominant philosophical ideas. There are many forms of the therapy, but all aim to enhance the flow of prana via the chakras. In *Ashtanga yoga*, breathing is synchronized with the postures increasing the purifying and strengthening qualities of the yoga practice. *Bhakti yoga* emphasizes selfless love and devotion. *Hatha yoga* is a forceful yoga used to purify and strengthen the body on its way to self enlightenment through asanas to restore and maintain well-being, increase vitality and flexibility and facilitate meditation. *Iyengar yoga* is characterized by precision and attention to detail, particularly in relation to the correct alignment of the body. *Karma yoga* is based on outward sacrifice and inward meditation and is the spiritual arm of yoga with the aim of attaining personal self realization. *Kundalini yoga* is a combination of coordinating postures, breathing, chanting and meditation aimed to awaken the 'serpent power' within the body, thus leading to spiritual emergence. *Mantra yoga* uses sonic vibrations to unify consciousness through recitation and contemplation of special sounds such as OM intended to elicit specific vibrational effects. *Nidra yoga* aids progressive relaxation of mind and body culminating in the 'corpse pose' and release of emotional tension. *Patanjalis yoga* aims for self realization and self knowledge. *Polarity yoga* involves stretches, sound and movement used in combination with other interventions during polarity therapy. *Raja yoga* is organized into eight aspects to purify mind and body. *Sivananda yoga* incorporates mantras and meditation, with an emphasis on breathing and relaxation.

Evidence:    There is considerable evidence of the value of yoga for a range of health issues including ageing-related conditions such as menopause and diabetes, for stress-related problems including headache, anxiety and depression and for other clinical fields such as maternity care.

Safety:    Certain postures are not advisable for those with hypertension, cardiac pathology and pregnant women. Many yoga sessions finish with a relaxation period which would be contraindicated in acute psychotic states or for those susceptible to psychosis. Caution if meditation is included in the session, trance-like states can lead to feelings of disorientation and depersonalization and should not be entered into for long periods. Emotional abreaction may occur. The varying philosophies and styles of yoga suggest that those intending to take up the practice should ensure the style they choose fits with their own personal philosophy.

Bibliography

Bhatia R, Dureja G P, Tripathi M et al 2007 Role of temporalis muscle over activity in chronic tension type headache: effect of yoga based management. Indian Journal of Physiology and Pharmacology 51(4):333–344

Butler L D, Waelde L C, Hastings T A et al 2008 Meditation with yoga, group therapy with hypnosis, and psychoeducation for long-term depressed mood: a randomized pilot trial. Journal of Clinical Psychology 64(7):806–820

Chattha R, Raghuram N, Venkatram P et al 2008 Treating the climacteric symptoms in Indian women with an integrated approach to yoga therapy: a randomized control study. Menopause 6 May [Epub ahead of print]

Chuntharapat S, Petpichetchian W, Hatthakit U 2008 Yoga during pregnancy: effects on maternal comfort, labor pain and birth outcomes. Complementary Therapies in Clinical Practice 14(2):105–115

Gordon L A, Morrison E Y, McGrowder D A et al 2008 Effect of exercise therapy on lipid profile and oxidative stress indicators in patients with type 2 diabetes. BMC Complementary and Alternative Medicine 8:21

Lipton L 2008 Using yoga to treat disease: an evidence-based review. Journal of the American Academy of Physician Assistants 21(2):34–36, Comment: 38, 41

Smith C, Hancock H, Blake-Mortimer J et al 2007 A randomised comparative trial of yoga and relaxation to reduce stress and anxiety. Complementary Therapies in Medicine 15(2):77–83

### Resources

British Wheel of Yoga: www.bwy.org.uk

Yoga Biomedical Trust/Yoga Therapy Centre: www.yogatherapy.org

## Urine therapy/urotherapy/uropathy

Drinking a midstream specimen of urine is deemed to be laxative in Ayurvedic medicine and the practice of drinking urine has a long history. It is mentioned on the Ebers Papyri of Ancient Egypt and the therapy was endorsed by Hippocrates. It is reported to slow the ageing process and is thought to improve mood. A midstream specimen is drunk first thing in the morning.

Evidence:   No studies to support this therapy were found.

Safety: No information regarding safety and no evidence of contraindications was found. Care should be taken regarding the sterility of the specimen.

### Bibliography

No professional literature found.

# Japanese medicine/kampo

Japan's traditional system of medicine evolved from traditional Chinese medicine (TCM, see examples below) and is based on similar principles of re-balancing chi (*ki* in Japanese), but which has also developed its own emphasis, integrated with Shinto and Buddhist philosophy. Modern day practitioners must, under Japanese law, be western-trained doctors or pharmacists. Diagnosis is similar to TCM but techniques vary; treatment aims to restore and maintain homeostasis and address issues related to the environment. Treatment may include diet using balancing foods from land, sea and mountain, breathing and exercise, shiatsu, acupuncture, herbal medicine (*kampo*), energy healing such as reiki and other therapies such as hydrotherapy to treat deficient or excessive ki. Massage is also used, including *anma* which involves stretching, squeezing and massaging to stimulate to restore and maintain good health, through improving muscle condition, influencing the internal organs and re-balancing ki; *ampuku*, which is a form of abdominal massage, used both for diagnosis and treatment; and *johrei*, which aims to remove toxins from the body through touch and to promote a more natural way of life, which is particularly useful for stress-related conditions, allergies and chronic pain.

Evidence:    There are reviews, reports and some formal research studies on the effectiveness of kampo for a range of medical conditions, including headache, premenstrual syndrome, menopause, rheumatoid arthritis and cancer.

Safety:    Concern has been expressed over the possible interactions between Japanese kampo and conventional drugs.

---

### Bibliography

Efferth T, Miyachi H, Bartsch H 2007 Pharmacogenomics of a traditional Japanese herbal medicine (Kampo) for cancer therapy. Cancer Genomics and Proteomics 4(2):81–91

Makino T, Mizuno F, Mizukami H 2006 Does a kampo medicine containing schisandra fruit affect pharmacokinetics of nifedipine like grapefruit juice? Biological and Pharmaceutical Bulletin 29(10):2065–2069

Ogawa K, Kojima T, Matsumoto C et al 2007 Identification of a predictive biomarker for the beneficial effect of a Kampo (Japanese traditional) medicine keishibukuryogan in rheumatoid arthritis patients. Clinical Biochemistry 40(15):1113–1121

Pan B, Kato Y, Sengoku K et al 2004 Treatment of climacteric symptoms with herbal formulas of traditional Chinese medicine. Gynecologic and Obstetric Investigation 57(3):144–148

Toyoshima M, Chida K, Suda T et al 2008 A case of pneumonitis caused by Seisin-renshi-in, herbal medicine. Nihon Kokyuki Gakkai Zasshi 46(1):31–34, [in Japanese]

Yamada K, Kanba S 2007 Effectiveness of kamishoyosan for premenstrual dysphoric disorder: open-labeled pilot study. Psychiatry and Clinical Neuroscience 61(3):323–325

## Reiki

Developed by the Japanese Dr Mikao Usui, reiki is a hands-on method of channelling the universal life energy from one person to another to restore internal harmony and release physical, mental or spiritual blockages. The practitioner attunes and places his hands on the patient, with fingers together, so that energy is transferred from giver to recipient, releasing tension and increasing blood flow, the hand positions corresponding with the chakras of Ayurvedic medicine. Treatment finishes with myofascial techniques and effleurage to close the energy channels.

Evidence:    There appears to be little formal literature on the Japanese form of reiki, although there is considerable evidence for Therapeutic Touch, as practised in the USA. Reports on reiki found when searching the literature are primarily published in western journals, by practitioners who have isolated the use of reiki as a modality in its own right, rather than as a component of Japanese traditional medicine. Reiki appears to have been used for pain relief and relaxation but whether this is due to a placebo effect is difficult to determine.

Safety:    Contraindicated over open wounds or factures, some patients may be aware of the energetic shift, which may cause discomfort.

Bibliography

Potter P J 2007 Breast biopsy and distress: feasibility of testing a Reiki intervention. Journal of Holistic Nursing 25(4):238–248

Raingruber B, Robinson C 2007 The effectiveness of Tai Chi, yoga, meditation and Reiki healing sessions in promoting health and enhancing problem solving abilities of registered nurses. Issues in Mental Health Nursing 28(10):1141–1155

Sharma V G, Sanghvi C, Mehta Y et al 2000 Efficacy of reiki on patients undergoing coronary artery bypass graft surgery. Annals of Cardiac Anaesthesia 3(2):12–18

Resources

UK Reiki Federation: www.reikifed.co.uk

*Shiatsu*

Shiatsu (meaning 'thumb pressure') is a modern version of anma, developed in the mid-20th century, in which the practitioner uses thumbs, arms and knees to stimulate pressure points along the meridians, stimulating the musculoskeletal system and inducing a feeling of deep mental relaxation. Diagnosis includes taking a history, observation, smelling, listening and palpating. There are several variations of shiatsu including *namikoshi*, which concentrates on physical techniques developed from anma, drawing on Western knowledge of anatomy and physiology and focusing less on the traditional concepts of meridians and Yin and Yang balance; *tsubo* therapy, which is based on research into the electrical resistance of the skin over tsubo (acupuncture) points and involves tsubo stimulation through massage, needles, electrical devices and moxa; *Zen shiatsu* which blends amna with the concepts of Yin and Yang, ki and meridian theory, including the five element theory and in which the whole meridian is worked, not just the relevant tsubos or acupressure points.

Evidence: There are numerous reports of successful alleviation of sickness, of various aetiologies, from stimulation of the pericardium 6 tsubo, although this could be classified under acupressure as opposed to shiatsu. Similarly, pressure applied to other points has been successful in relieving fatigue during chemotherapy and easing trauma pain and the effects of dementia in the elderly. Precise stimulation of shiatsu points has also been used to trigger uterine contractions in expectant mothers past their expected date of delivery.

Safety: Prolonged use can lead to nerve and arterial damage.

Bibliography

Can Gürkan O, Arslan H 2008 Effect of acupressure on nausea and vomiting during pregnancy. Complementary Therapies in Clinical Practice 14(1):46–52

Ingram J, Domagala C, Yates S 2005 The effects of shiatsu on post-term pregnancy. Complementary Therapies in Medicine 13(1):11–15

Lang T, Hager H, Funovits V et al 2007 Prehospital analgesia with acupressure at the Baihui and Hegu points in patients with radial fractures: a prospective, randomized, double-blind trial. American Journal of Emergency Medicine 25(8): 887–893

Molassiotis A, Sylt P, Diggins H 2007 The management of cancer-related fatigue after chemotherapy with acupuncture and acupressure: a randomised controlled trial. Complementary Therapies in Medicine 15(4):228–237

Perkins P, Vowler S L 2008 Does acupressure help reduce nausea and vomiting in palliative care patients? Pilot study. Palliative Medicine 22(2):193–194

Shin H S, Song Y A, Seo S 2007 Effect of Nei-Guan point (P6) acupressure on ketonuria levels, nausea and vomiting in women with hyperemesis gravidarum. Journal of Advanced Nursing 59(5):510–519

Yang M H, Wu S C, Lin J G et al 2007 The efficacy of acupressure for decreasing agitated behaviour in dementia: a pilot study. Journal of Clinical Nursing 16(2):308–315

---

### Resources

---

Shiatsu Society: www.shiatsu.org

## Traditional Chinese medicine (TCM)

*Description*

TCM is an integrated medical system developed in China, approximately 2500 years ago, but now used throughout Asia. It is based on the notion that humans have a vital force or life energy (*Qi*), which flows around the body via 12 major energy channels, called meridians, linking one part of the body to another; along the meridians are over 2000 focus points called tsubos or acupoints. Imbalances, as a result of disease or ill-health, may present as excess or deficient energy (Qi) or stasis, caused by internal factors such as the *seven emotions* (anger, joy, sadness, grief, pensiveness, fear and fright) or external factors (*the six evils* – wind, cold, damp, fire and heat. Diagnosis is complex and involves inspection, tongue diagnosis; listening to breath and heart sounds; smelling of breath, body odour and excreta; a full medical history based on the sensations of hot and cold, perspiration, diet, excreta, headache, body aches, chest, thirst, previous illnesses and medications; palpation of acupuncture points and pulses; identification of patterns according to the eight principles of interior/exterior, hot/cold, full/empty and Yin/Yang; and patterns according to the five elements of wood, earth, water, fire and metal.

The concept of Yin and Yang is a naturalistic one based on early observation echoing aspects of the lunar cycle and the cycle of the seasons. Yang encompasses aspects of light, heaven, sun, day, spring, summer, hot, male, fast, upwards, outside, fire, wood. Yin encompasses aspects of dark, earth, moon, night, autumn, winter, cold, female, slow, downwards, inside, water, metal. The principle of TCM is to maintain the balance of Yin/Yang through tonifying Yang or Yin and/or eliminating excess Yang or Yin, as appropriate. In *five element theory*, it is thought that the universe comprises five elements – Water, Fire, Wood, Metal and Earth – which are in a state of perpetual movement, interacting with each other. These five states each relate to an aspect of the human body, enabling effective diagnosis and treatment in accordance with the state of the outside world. Treatment aims to treat disease from the root cause and eliminate evil influences (external pathogens); it incorporates dietary modifications based on analysis of the individuals' tastes, including sour, bitter, sweet, pungent and salty flavours, exercise such as tai chi and qi gong, massage, acupuncture, moxibustion, cupping and herbal medicine in order to re-balance disharmonies within the body's Qi.

Evidence:   Most reviews and published research studies are in Chinese, intimating that methodology may not be as rigorous as in the west and some sweeping claims for efficacy are made in some papers, from the results of single case studies. However, there is an increasing number of papers in English, with some promising suggestions for the effectiveness of various aspects of TCM, notably some of the herbal remedies and in particular, acupuncture.

Safety:   There have been several sensational reports in the western media of toxicity from herbal remedies imported from China, significantly hepatic failure: patients with liver disease should be advised to avoid Chinese herbal preparations.

## Bibliography

Chen F P, Kung Y Y, Chen Y C et al 2008 Frequency and pattern of Chinese herbal medicine prescriptions for chronic hepatitis in Taiwan. Journal of Ethnopharmacology 117(1):84–91

Cheng H Y, Huang H H, Yang C M et al 2008 The in vitro anti-herpes simplex virus type-1 and type-2 activity of Long Dan Xie Gan Tan, a prescription of traditional chinese medicine. Chemotherapy 54(2):77–83

Fei Y T, Liu J P 2008 Herbal CONSORT statement and standardization of reporting traditional. Chinese drug trials Zhongguo Zhong Yao Za Zhi 33(1):89–94 [in Chinese]

Langmead L, Rampton D S 2001 Review article: herbal treatment in gastrointestinal and liver disease: benefits and dangers. Alimentary Pharmacology and Therapeutics 15(9):1239–1252

McRae C A, Agarwal K, Mutimer D et al 2002 Hepatitis associated with Chinese herbs. European Journal of Gastroenterology and Hepatology 14(5):559–562

Rong J, Cheung C Y, Lau A S et al 2008 Induction of heme oxygenase-1 by traditional Chinese medicine formulation ISF-1 and its ingredients as a cytoprotective mechanism against oxidative stress. International Journal of Molecular Medicine 21(4):405–411

Wang L, Zhou G B, Liu P et al 2008 Dissection of mechanisms of Chinese medicinal formula Realgar-Indigo naturalis as an effective treatment for promyelocytic leukemia. Proceedings of the National Academy of Science U S A 105(12):4826–4831

## Resources

Foundation for Traditional Chinese Medicine: www.ftcm.org.uk

### Acupuncture

Acupuncture is one of several TCM treatment modalities in which needles are inserted into identified tsubos (acupoints) in order to re-balance the Qi. A sensation of distension, aching, heaviness, tingling, warmth, soreness or numbness felt by the patient around the area of acupuncture needle insertion (termed *deqi*), indicates that the needles have been inserted to a therapeutically effective depth. Numbness is thought to be produced by stimulation of large diameter A beta fibres and heaviness by stimulation of large diameter A delta fibres.

Different forms of acupuncture include: electro-acupuncture, laser acupuncture, which uses low emission laser beams instead of needles and auricular acupuncture, in which the ear is viewed as a micro-system of the body with points identified on it and stimulated in the same way as full body acupuncture. Acupressure uses finger or thumb pressure at the relevant points and can be effective for people averse to needles, including children. Trigger point acupuncture is a western modification, in which needles inserted into specific trigger points (foci of neural hyperactivity which refer pain to adjacent or distant structures) are used primarily to relieve referred pain; it does not comply with the holistic principles of classical acupuncture of TCM. Acupuncture has been used for analgesia – it has been shown that insertion of acupuncture needles, sometimes electrically charged, triggers release of endorphins which inhibit or modify the transmission of pain signals. Neurotransmitters involved include: dopamine, noradrenalin and somatostatin and serotonin.

Evidence: There are numerous studies, of good calibre, on the effectiveness of acupuncture for a wide range of medical conditions and symptoms, including gynaecological orthopaedic, gastrointestinal and critical care patients. Acupressure has also been shown to be effective for nausea and vomiting and a commercial wristband (Seabands™) is available in the UK for self-stimulation of the pericardium 6 acupoint.

Safety: Caution regarding patients with bleeding disorders or on anticoagulants. Fainting or dizziness can occur during treatment as a result of hypotension. Although rare, some individuals may be allergic to the metal of the needles, leading to the development of localized rashes. Infection at the site of needles insertion could be a risk if unsterilized needles are used, but this should not normally be a problem when the practitioner is a professionally trained clinical acupuncturist. Reactions to acupuncture can vary, so caution with concurrent medication for referred problem.

## Bibliography

Berkovitz S, Cummings M, Perrin C et al 2008 High volume acupuncture clinic (HVAC) for chronic knee pain: audit of a possible model for delivery of acupuncture in the National Health Service. Acupuncture in Medicine 26(1):46–50

Cherkin D C, Sherman K J, Hogeboom C J et al 2008 Efficacy of acupuncture for chronic low back pain: protocol for a randomized controlled trial. Trials 9:10

Ee C C, Manheimer E, Pirotta M V et al 2008 Acupuncture for pelvic and back pain in pregnancy: a systematic review. American Journal of Obstetrics and Gynecology 198(3):254–259

Frisk J, Carlhäll S, Källström A C et al 2008 Long-term follow-up of acupuncture and hormone therapy on hot flushes in women with breast cancer: a prospective, randomized, controlled multicenter trial. Climacteric 11(2):166–174

McDonough S M, Liddle S D, Hunter R et al 2008 Exercise and manual auricular acupuncture: a pilot assessor-blind randomised controlled trial. BMC Musculoskeletal Disorders 9(1):31

Nayak S, Wenstone R, Jones A et al 2008 Surface electrostimulation of acupuncture points for sedation of critically ill patients in the intensive care unit: a pilot study. Acupuncture in Medicine 26(1):1–7

Reynolds J A, Bland J M, Macpherson H 2008 Acupuncture for irritable bowel syndrome an exploratory randomised controlled trial. Acupuncture in Medicine 26(1):8–16

Witt C M, Reinhold T, Jena S et al 2008 Cost-effectiveness of acupuncture treatment in patients with headache. Cephalalgia 28(4):334–345

## Resources

British Acupuncture Council (BAcC): www.acupuncture.org.uk
British Medical Acupuncture Society (BMAS): www.medical-acupuncture.co.uk
Acupuncture Association of Chartered Physiotherapists (AACP): www.aacp.uk.com

## Cupping

Cupping is a TCM technique, in which a warmed glass cup is placed over an area of congestion or an acupuncture point in order to create a vacuum, with the aim of withdrawing excess Qi.

Evidence: There appears to be limited research evidence specifically on the procedure of cupping. Its effectiveness in treating various conditions has been demonstrated in a number of Chinese studies, although these are often in combination with other aspects of TCM, including acupuncture and herbal remedies, an the majority of papers are published in Chinese language journals.

Safety: The primary risk from cupping appears to be the danger of burns when combined with the burning of Chinese herbs.

## Bibliography

Ahmadi A, Schwebel D C, Rezaei M 2008 The efficacy of wet-cupping in the treatment of tension and migraine headache. American Journal of Chinese Medicine 36(1):37–44

Chen S 2007 The clustered needling, massage and cupping used for treatment of obstinate myofascitis of the back: a report of 68 cases. Journal of Traditional Chinese Medicine 27(2):113–114

Iblher N, Stark B 2007 Cupping treatment and associated burn risk: a plastic surgeon's perspective. Journal of Burn Care and Research 28(2):355–358

Lüdtke R, Albrecht U, Stange R et al 2006 Brachialgia paraesthetica nocturna can be relieved by 'wet cupping' – results of a randomised pilot study. Complementary Therapies in Medicine 14(4):247–253

Niasari M, Kosari F, Ahmadi A 2007 The effect of wet cupping on serum lipid concentrations of clinically healthy young men: a randomized controlled trial. Journal of Alternative and Complementary Medicine 13(1):79–82

Tian J 2007 Electroacupuncture combined with flash cupping for treatment of peripheral facial paralysis: a report of 224 cases. Journal of Traditional Chinese Medicine 27(1):14–15

## Exercise

Various types of exercise are encouraged as part of TCM, including Qi gong, tai chi, meditation and breathing, fitness training and martial arts. Qi gong includes motor control, postural awareness, relaxation, breath control, visualization and meditation. Tai chi chuan is a dynamic form of Qi gong consisting of a programme of slow, controlled movements. It has become popular in the west as a gentle form of exercise and has been shown to be effective in improving a variety of symptoms, particularly in the elderly and for menopausal symptoms.

Evidence: There is considerable evidence of the value of tai chi, Qi gong and other slow movement and exercise techniques employed within TCM, for patients with mobility-limiting conditions, including Parkinson's disease and in the elderly and in menopausal women.

Safety: Tai chi can induce deep relaxation therefore contraindicated for patients with psychosis or hallucinations but may benefit the patient during a non-active period of illness; a psychotic episode has been reported in one woman practising qi gong.

### Bibliography

Aickin M 2007 Does T'ai Chi Chuan improve health-related quality of life in elderly patients? Journal of Alternative and Complementary Medicine 13(10):1053

Chang Y F, Yang Y H, Chen C C et al 2008 Tai Chi Chuan training improves the pulmonary function of asthmatic children. Journal of Microbiology, Immunology and Infection 41(1):88–95

Hackney M E, Earhart G M 2008 Tai Chi improves balance and mobility in people with Parkinson disease. Gait Posture 28(3):456–460

Lansinger B, Larsson E, Persson L C et al 2007 Qigong and exercise therapy in patients with long-term neck pain: a prospective randomized trial. Spine 32(22):2415–2422

Hwang W C 2007 Qi-gong psychotic reaction in a Chinese American woman. Culture, Medicine and Psychiatry 31(4):547–560

Lui P P, Qin L, Chan K M 2008 Tai Chi Chuan exercises in enhancing bone mineral density in active seniors. Clinical Sports Medicine 27(1):75–86

Mariano C 2008 A 16-week tai chi programme prevented falls in healthy older adults. Evidence Based Nursing 11(2):60

Pei Y C, Chou S W, Lin P S et al 2008 Eye-hand coordination of elderly people who practice Tai Chi Chuan. Journal of the Formosan Medical Association 107(2):103–110

Yu W L, Li X Q, Tang W J et al 2007 fMRI study of pain reaction in the brain under state of 'Qigong'. American Journal of Chinese Medicine 35(6):937–945

*Chinese herbal medicine*

A variety of indigenous plants are used in TCM to re-balance the flow of Qi, administered orally in teas and tinctures, dermally via compresses and poultices and occasionally via other routes. They often taste unusual or unpleasant when first ingested but the taste improves as the patient's condition improves. Herbs are commonly prescribed in combinations of up to 15 herbs, there being nearly 6000 herbs available to qualified practitioners, plus some animal and mineral ingredients. In the west, Chinese herbal medicine is most often used to treat skin disease, allergies, digestive, gynaecological, respiratory and immune system problems, as well as pain and addiction.

Evidence: There is little English-language research evidence of good calibre and many of the Chinese papers are single case repots. Sensational media reports of fatal contaminants found in imported Chinese herbal medicines has done little to improve credibility in the west.

Safety: The chemical constituents of Chinese herbal medicines are diverse and there is little evidence available in the West regarding safety or potential toxicity. Dose limitations are applied, although this may be significantly more than the approved dose for similar substances used in the West, e.g. the maximum daily dose of ginger in the West is considered to be 1 g, whereas in China, up to 3 g daily may be used. Some Chinese herbal products may interact with each other and many interact with conventional pharmacological medication. Concern continues over the import of unlicensed herbal preparations, with blends of unknown constituents and there have been reports of serious side-effects such as lead poisoning, from contaminated batches brought into the UK and USA, one of the justifications for classifying TCM in Group 3 of the House of Lords Report on Complementary Medicine (2000).

Bibliography

Dengfeng W, Taixiang W, Lina H et al 2007 Chinese herbal medicines in the treatment of ectopic pregnancy. Cochrane Database of Systematic Reviews(4), Comment: CD006224

Gu C L, Zhang Y K, Fu Y X et al 2007 Effect of tiaozhi yanggan decoction in treating patients with non-alcoholic fatty liver. Chinese Journal of Integrative Medicine 13(4):275–279

Miller G M, Stripp R 2007 A study of western pharmaceuticals contained within samples of Chinese herbal/patent medicines collected from New York City's Chinatown. Legal Medicine (Tokyo, Japan) 9(5):258–264

Yong E L, Wong S P, Shen P et al 2007 Standardization and evaluation of botanical mixtures: lessons from a traditional Chinese herb, Epimedium, with oestrogenic properties. Novartis Foundation Symposium 282:173–188

### Chinese massage

Various types of massage and manual techniques are incorporated into TCM, including *anmo*, which means 'pressing and rubbing' and involves manipulations, traction and stretching. Anmo is a precursor to *tui na*, which means 'pushing and pulling' and involves soft tissue massage, rolling, gliding, kneading and percussion, based on the principles of meridian work and harmonizing of the Yin/Yang balance. Daoyin is a self-administered programme of massage, breathing, meditation and stretching exercises, which aims to eliminate toxins, promote self development and increase spirituality.

Evidence:   There appears to be little published evidence specifically on the manual techniques employed in TCM, apart from acupressure and acupuncture, unless used in combination with other aspects of TCM. Almost all papers found were in Chinese.

Safety:   Avoid in fractures, open lesions, osteoporosis and infections. Avoid lower back and abdominal massage during pregnancy. As with any manual therapy, caution should be taken following surgery or injury, during pregnancy and postpartum. If the patient is recovering from injury or illness or is in a rehabilitation programme, suggest they discuss the therapy with physiotherapist or specialist.

Bibliography

Du D 2007 Treatment of prolapse of lumbar intervertebral disc by tuina massotherapy combined with oral administration of buyang huanwu tang: a report of 75 cases. Journal of Traditional Chinese Medicine 27(1):43–45

Dune L 2006 Integrating tuina acupressure and traditional Chinese medicine concepts into a holistic nursing practice. Explore (NY) 2(6):543–546

### Moxibustion

Moxibustion, sometimes called acu-moxa therapy, involves burning dried artemesia leaves directly or indirectly over relevant acupuncture points to re-balance Qi. Most commonly 'moxa rolls' are lit, the flame is quenched and the smoking stick is positioned 2 cm away from the skin, but in some cases moxa is applied directly to the skin, producing a scar or blister. Acupuncture needles may be inserted and the moxa applied to the handle and ignited, warming the needle. Moxibustion is used as a heat source to stimulate deficient Qi and has become extremely popular in the West, as an alternative treatment for correcting breech presentation in pregnancy.

Evidence: Most papers on moxibustion are in Chinese, but the increasing interest in using the technique to turn breech-presenting fetuses to cephalic has spawned a number of good quality studies, published in English language journals. Abstracts viewed from Chinese papers suggest that moxibustion has various positive effects and is a valuable component of TCM.

Safety: The main risk is from burns: patients whose manual dexterity is impaired should not self-administer moxibustion. Those with hypertension should avoid moxibustion. In maternity care, midwives should advise mothers wishing to use moxibustion as an alternative to external cephalic version or caesarean section for breech presentation to ensure that the practitioner whom they consult is adequately trained to identify exclusion criteria (e.g. low lying placenta, previous uterine scar, multiple pregnancy).

### Bibliography

Cardini F, Lombardo P, Regalia A L et al 2005 A randomised controlled trial of moxibustion for breech presentation. British Journal of Obstetrics and Gynaecology 112(6):743–747

Chau N 2006 Moxibustion burns. Journal of Hospital Medicine 1(6):367

Choi G S, Han J B, Park J H et al 2004 Effects of moxibustion to zusanli (ST36) on alteration of natural killer cell activity in rats. American Journal of Chinese Medicine 32(2):303–312

Guo J 2007 Chronic fatigue syndrome treated by acupuncture and moxibustion in combination with psychological approaches in 310 cases. Journal of Traditional Chinese Medicine 27(2):92–95

Joos S, Wildau N, Kohnen R et al 2006 Acupuncture and moxibustion in the treatment of ulcerative colitis: a randomized controlled study. Scandinavian Journal of Gastroenterology 41(9):1056–1063

Konkimalla V B, Efferth T 2008 Evidence-based Chinese medicine for cancer therapy. Journal of Ethnopharmacology 116(2):207–210

Neri I, De Pace V, Venturini P et al 2007 Effects of three different stimulations (acupuncture, moxibustion, acupuncture plus moxibustion) of BL.67 acupoint at small toe on fetal behavior of breech presentation. American Journal of Chinese Medicine 35(1):27–33

Sakakibara R, Murakami E, Katagiri A et al 2007 Moxibustion, an alternative therapy, ameliorated disturbed circadian rhythm of plasma arginine vasopressin and urine output in multiple system atrophy. Internal Medicine (Tokyo, Japan) 46(13):1015–1018

Wang T, Zhang Q, Xue X et al 2008 A systematic review of acupuncture and moxibustion treatment for chronic fatigue syndrome in china. American Journal of Chinese Medicine 36(1):1–24

Yun S P, Jung W S, Park S U et al 2007 Effects of moxibustion on the recovery of post-stroke urinary symptoms. American Journal of Chinese Medicine 35(6):947–954